STOP AGING START TRAINING

Look and Feel Twenty Years Younger

Salvatore Fichera, M.S.

D1502435

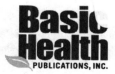

Basic Health
PUBLICATIONS, INC.

The information contained in this book is based upon the research and personal and professional experiences of the author. It is not intended as a substitute for consulting with your physician or other healthcare provider. Any attempt to diagnose and treat an illness should be done under the direction of a healthcare professional.

The publisher does not advocate the use of any particular healthcare protocol but believes the information in this book should be available to the public. The publisher and author are not responsible for any adverse effects or consequences resulting from the use of the suggestions, preparations, or procedures discussed in this book. Should the reader have any questions concerning the appropriateness of any procedures or preparation mentioned, the author and the publisher strongly suggest consulting a professional healthcare advisor.

Basic Health Publications, Inc.
28812 Top of the World Drive
Laguna Beach, CA 92651
949-715-7327 • www.basichealthpub.com

Library of Congress Cataloging-in-Publication Data

Fichera, Salvatore
    Stop aging, start training : look and feel twenty years younger / Salvatore Fichera.
      p. cm.
    Includes bibliographical references.
    ISBN 978-1-59120-218-9
 1. Physical fitness. 2. Longevity. I. Title.

    RA781.F495   2008
    613.7—dc22

                                     2008020744

Editor: Roberta W. Waddell
Typesetting/Book design: Gary A. Rosenberg
Cover design: Mike Stromberg
Exercise Photos: Salvatore Fichera

Printed in the United States of America

10   9   8   7   6   5   4   3   2   1

Contents

PART TWO
Exercises:
Applications and Illustrations

This book is dedicated to my wife, Ryoko,
and my mom, Katherine.

Ryoko has had the never-ending patience that any man would
want in a woman. Whether it's late nights at the gym (until
midnight, many times) or for Saturdays devoted to my writing,
she never questions my lengthy hours of work. I am grateful
for her unending love, support, understanding . . . and faith.

Since childhood, my mom has been a source of inspiration—
a role model who has endlessly set examples for how a healthy,
active lifestyle can slow down, or reverse, the effects of aging.
She made me realize how the number that represents age
does not represent a person's youthfulness. She, too, has
endlessly supported me emotionally and spiritually in
all my endeavors, always keeping her faith in
my success and her love unconditional.

Acknowledgments

If I were to thank all the people who have helped me—directly and indirectly—through their inspiration, friendship, and education, I would need to devote an entire chapter to the acknowledgments.

So with the available space, I would specifically like to thank the following people for their contributions and assistance in making this book a reality.

Ryoko Maebayashi-Fichera, who is not only my soulmate, but also an excellent photo assistant.

Katherine Fichera, who, in addition to being a fantastic mom, role model, and best friend, was an exercise model.

Carmela Fichera, who, in addition to being a wonderful sister, was also an exercise model.

Richard Fichera, my dad, who was not a model, but a role model in being a hard worker and a dedicated family man.

Arlene Uslander and Rusty Fischer, for their exceptional editorial guidance.

Paul Auerbach, for being a long-time friend and exercise model for this book.

Irini Rez, for being readily available to assist me, whether as an exercise model for my website and this book, or for presenting a TV news report on health.

Florence Chan and Susan Winter, for being exercise models in the first round of photographs, which unfortunately do not appear in this book.

Gold's Gym owners, for allowing me to use their downtown John Street facility to showcase the exercises in this book.

José Herrera, night manager of Gold's Gym, NYC, for allowing me to hold the photo shoots after the club was closed for the night.

The entire Queens College (CUNY) staff of Ph.D.s and professors in exercise physiology—namely Dr. McArdle and Dr. Toner—for their skillful teaching, insight, and knowledge of this field I love with such passion.

Peggy Sirdula, client, friend, and artist, who spent an enormous amount of time detailing the figures on page 39.

Norm Goldfind, for hearing my message and granting me the opportunity to publish this book. Bobby Waddell, my editor, and Gary Rosenberg, the book's designer, for being such a great, supportive team. Diane Glynn, for her assistance in promoting my book.

Introduction

Age. It's something none of us can avoid. Every year we get a little older, a little more tired, a little less inclined to move. Being active becomes a chore, eating less requires more effort, and every day some new diet that promises *guaranteed results* is guaranteed to do only one thing—disappoint us.

But does it *have* to be this way?

Regardless of your age, would you like to have more energy, an increased sex drive, and look your absolute best? Would you like to feel better than you did last year? The year before? Heck, would you like to feel better at forty-five, fifty-five, sixty-five, seventy-five, or even eighty-five than you did at thirty-five? Or even twenty-five?

Well, it's possible because we *can* stop, and even reverse, the aging process. The fitness and nutritional guidelines detailed in this book can help Baby Boomers (and anyone else) look and feel ten to twenty years younger. *Strength training* is central to this process, and it's one of the most direct ways of attaining and maintaining a youthful existence. If the words strength training frighten you, the good news is that it's easy to begin such a program and, better yet, it can start from the privacy and convenience of your own home.

To illustrate my point, stop reading for a moment and stand up. (Trust me, it's worth it.) When you reach a fully straightened position, pause, and then slowly come back to the seated position. Just now, you performed one full repetition of an exercise called *squats*. (Congratulations. Keep it up, and this book can pay for itself by page 10.) "So," I can hear you asking, "What's a squat? And why should I keep squatting?"

Squats challenge your front and back thighs and buttocks. Now do this

1

movement eleven more times and you will have completed a full set . . . and already you will be on your way to becoming stronger and younger.

That's right. You don't need gyms or expensive equipment to embark on a quest for youthful living. At this stage, all you need is *determination* . . . and, of course, professional guidance. That's where this book can help. In it, I will take you by the hand and guide you step by step to a more youthful, vigorous, and healthy future.

The exercise programs here have done a great deal for me personally, and they have dramatically changed the lives of my clients for two decades. Now I want to share them with you. And I am sure that, by sticking with these programs, you will love the results—the new you—all starting in as little as four weeks. That's one month to a livelier, more energetic, youthful you.

Despite the abundance of fitness books on the market today, none have addressed *all* the significant elements needed for success. Books targeting older populations, in particular, tend to come up short when it comes to addressing the three most important components of exercise: *variety, proper technique,* and *intensity.* By contrast, not only does *Stop Aging—Start Training* cover how to exercise, but it also offers the most complete discussion of these three elements on the market. This thought-provoking, powerfully candid tool for reawakening both physical and mental values:

- Is written in an easy-to-implement style utilizing an Action Plan designed to be read in easy-to-digest, educational, entertaining capsules.

- Is written in everyday language, to encourage members of all socio-economic levels.

- Provides a direct and measurable physical benefit in *improved, more youthful health.*

- Is both entertaining and informative, and is peppered with my personal anecdotes as an exercise physiologist, professional speaker, and certified personal trainer.

- Contains the motivation, inspiration, and *information* needed to create a healthier, happier population.

- Is packed with concrete advice to use every single day that will inspire you to feel good, look great, and live longer—no matter what your age.

- Is a solid learning tool—factual, believable, inspirational, and enjoyable to read.

Is This Book for You?

You bet it is. *Stop Aging—Start Training* is written for Baby Boomers (or anyone who has begun to notice their body is aging) interested in living a longer, stronger, and happier life. While directed at both genders, women in particular will benefit from this book as they are more susceptible to osteoporosis and are typically more concerned about fat accumulation (in addition to being more prone to it). As readers will find, both of these issues are directly controllable through strength training.

A very unique feature of this book is that it is like an invisible hand guiding you from your couch to your exercise station—whether that means the living room floor, a mat in the garage, a Swiss ball, or the gym. This book will take you from being *sedentary,* to becoming *active,* to living more *youthfully.* All in *four* short weeks.

Feeling skeptical? Feel like you've been left out of the exercise/diet-book loop? The following seven points help make *Stop Aging—Start Training* a more effective, user-friendly tool for you to implement into your own lifestyle. It has:

1. A greater variety of exercises than is offered by other such books.

2. Detailed exercise descriptions and photos, helping you to easily master the techniques.

3. Detailed program options so that, regardless of your current fitness level, you can begin comfortably at your appropriate level of intensity.

4. Thorough discussions about which portion of muscles is being targeted by each exercise, rather than mere mentions of general muscle groups. This helps you to target specific areas more easily.

5. Complete coverage of exercise sequencing, the optimal sequential order in which exercises should be performed (an often-overlooked, critical element).

6. In-depth coverage of abs, lower-back flexibility, and core strength development. This is essential, since the core is the center for balance and strength.

7. Extensive references from scientific journals.

This book stresses the belief that the human body should have come with an *Owner's Manual.* And this is it.

Stop Aging—Start Training consists of two sections, plus the back matter. The first section is conceptual and theoretical, laying the groundwork for success in attaining health and fitness goals. The second section is practical, providing a full menu of exercises for each major muscle group, accompanied by detailed instructions and photographs. In back, there is a Glossary defining some of the less familiar terms in the book, followed by a list of Resources, a Reference section, and an Index.

A key element of this book is that no matter where you fall on the fitness scale, it will work for you. Why? Because it offers program options for three main levels of fitness—Beginner, Intermediate, and Advanced. The beginner section starts with a basic whole-body workout plan designed for first-timers, and the programs advance from there.

As a side note to what you may learn through the media, I feel the need to mention one thing. Every day, the media introduces new research, which presents an idea that may be completely contradictory to research presented in the recent past. Many times, the research quoted by media is merely at the stage where the idea is simply a hunch. Hungry for new stories, however, the media jumps on yet-to-be proven theories. The key is to avoid believing every single research item that comes out of scientific circles. Find out if such ideas are supported by numerous other studies.

Author's Note

Jack LaLanne, Canned Tomatoes, Bullies, and My Path to Lifelong Fitness

I was four-years-old, playing with my toy soldiers on the living room floor, just minding my own business. Suddenly, a man's voice boomed out of the TV and my mother leapt off the couch and began twisting herself like a pretzel, arms akimbo, legs splayed.

As the minutes passed and the TV man held court, her behavior got even more outlandish; with every cheerful command, she'd jump up and down . . . or run in place . . . or try to touch her toes. She'd hold cans of tomatoes over her head . . . hunch her shoulders up and down . . . roll her neck around . . . and breathe in, then puff out like a steam locomotive.

And always there was that familiar voice—encouraging, praising, cajoling. Maybe she told me the purpose of this madness once upon a time, but all I remember was being worried that she'd step on one of my precious toy soldiers. I didn't know at the time that this bundle-of-energy-guy who, like a Pied Piper, made my mother do pretzel contortions and canned tomato curls, was named Jack LaLanne (world-renowned fitness guru and host of the first-ever TV show on fitness, from 1951–1985) and I certainly didn't know the dramatic effect he was to have on my own life in years to come.

Eight years later, I was on the small side, and skinny. We lived in a tough working-class New York town and although this sounds like the awful ninety-seven-pound-weakling-cliché, I actually *was* getting shoved around by bullies on a daily basis.

After about two months of this abuse, however, I remembered that muscular TV-guy in tights who ordered my mother around, and how he was always talking about how you needed to exercise to get stronger. And so, at age twelve, I started doing pushups, chin-ups, and sit-ups. ("One, two, three," Jack would shout from our living room TV. "You can do it—one, two three.") Even though I really didn't know what I was doing, I did know it was time to start shoving back. The pushups seemed like a good place to start. If I could push up from the floor twenty or thirty times, shouldn't I be able to push a bully back at least *once*?

What started out as twenty-minutes twice a week slowly evolved into a daily routine of at least an hour. Even in the heat of summer, my determination to be better equipped for self-protection kept me going. (That, and the booming voice from our TV.)

It took a number of fistfights and bloody noses to prove my point. I transformed myself into a strong and fast fighter, no longer willing to accept bullying—even from the bigger guys. Picking on me was no longer fun—even if they thought they could win, they knew they were going to get hurt.

Looking back, I don't feel it was just the strength, but also my confidence that deterred those bullies. Maybe it was the way I walked or carried myself through the elementary school halls, but whatever the reason, the bullies simply began to leave me alone.

Next came high school. And girls. And another new obstacle. The jocks, with their strong, well-defined bodies, were attracting most of the girls. Once again, I remembered Jack and his muscles, and wondered if exercise could also make me more attractive to the opposite sex. So I put in the effort to shape and tone my body, this time just to look good. And it worked (at least, well enough).

I never minded the time it took to work out each day. I'd developed a routine of exercises that was comfortable for me and, though I pushed myself harder and harder each day, there was enough variety of movement to keep me interested, motivated, and disciplined.

The many payoffs didn't hurt, either. In college, looking good was still important, but other motivations began to emerge as I matured. I needed better endurance for sports, increased stamina for attending class, writing papers, and taking exams, etc. Not to mention going to the occasional party.

I also needed help with studying. Like many of my friends, I'd often crack the books late at night. But I'd just as often doze off, then wake up and hope to get some kind of second wind. This was a hit-and-miss philosophy, at best. One night, when I couldn't keep my eyes open any longer, however, I had a sudden inspiration from my mother's Jack LaLanne days. I dropped to the floor and did a few pushups. The first few reps were excruciating, I'd gone from sitting to sweating in sixty seconds, but then something amazing happened—the blood started pumping and the oxygen started flowing and my brain just seemed to perk up.

This was a terrific breakthrough for me and it was great to discover that whenever I felt overtired or unable to absorb any new information, exercise could jumpstart a mental second wind. So I continued to exercise regularly and found I was able to study longer, play sports harder, handle my school schedule better, and look pretty good in the bargain. Imagine that—four benefits from a single effort.

If only Wall Street paid out that many dividends for a single investment.

By age twenty-three, a career in real estate was burning me out. My life consisted of waking up, commuting, working a J.O.B. (which kept me Just Over Broke), commuting home, and then trying to recover from an endless stream of long, meaningless, monotonous days.

But once again, exercise would be my salvation. One Saturday in the summer of '87, I went to the beach for some soul-searching, and met three people jogging along the water line. On impulse, I joined them and we started to talk. One had recently graduated from college and mentioned that her major was exercise physiology (something I'd never heard of before—it was an epiphany of sorts for me). Then she excitedly told me about a job she was about to start. And after just a few minutes, all my dormant enthusiasm and passion resurfaced. As she talked, it suddenly became clear to me that I wanted to make exercise my profession, with the added bonus of teaching and helping others.

Fast-forward to today. It's now been over thirty-five years since I was last shoved by a bully, and exercise has taught me many physical, mental, and spiritual lessons. In the bargain, it has also taught me how to take control of my health, strength, and physique, and about the miraculous beauty of the perfectly designed, self-healing, and self-balancing human body.

This thing called exercise has taught me about self-discipline and how to apply it in any situation, be it personal, professional, physical, or mental. It has taught me how to diminish stress in all the most healthful ways, how to find happiness (even during difficult times), and it has helped me understand the interconnectedness between mind, body, and spirit.

And now that I am in my middle years, exercise has helped me to stay, look, and feel younger. There's no question about it: The older I get, the more numerous and varied the reasons I find for living a fit lifestyle.

Exercise has given me the opportunity to build a career I thoroughly enjoy—my work, in fact, feels more like play. And this all started with a TV show I never really watched. So thank you, Jack—you were the absolute best. And, of course, thank you Mom for being such an inspiration (and for not trampling my soldiers with your calisthenics and canned tomatoes).

Now it's your turn to find what motivates you to action. And with your motivation, we can work together toward creating a leaner, stronger, younger YOU!

Part One

The Complete Picture: Science, Ideas, and Philosophies

Whenever beginning a new endeavor, it is wise to first build a solid foundation—this is always the best first step. For *Stop Aging—Start Training,* this foundation includes nutrition, goal setting, and fitness assessments, as well as a discussion of the impact that being fit has on your life, both in terms of longevity and quality of life.

1

The Myths of Aging

Regardless of what your level of health and fitness knowledge is at present, chances are you've held a false viewpoint or engaged in ineffective, even dangerous exercise in the past. Unfortunately, this is an all too common and vicious cycle. Myths contribute to confusion, which, in turn, causes indecision. Indecision leads to inaction and the continuation of a sedentary lifestyle, which, in turn, causes more rapid aging. (Sound familiar?)

The first step toward halting the aging process, however, is to eliminate some of the major fallacies that prevent you from obtaining lifelong youthfulness and vitality. In other words, it's time to separate fact from fiction, myth from reality, age-causer from age-buster.

Having worked in the trenches (on the gym floor) nearly every week since 1987, I've heard every possible excuse, fallacy, and misconception pertaining to health and fitness that exists. Everything from: "I couldn't make it yesterday, my dog ate my leg warmers," to "The reason I think I've gained six pounds this week is because my toothpaste has too many calories."

Unfortunately, many crazed ideas and opinions originate from books and, in some cases, the popular and invasive media. It's human nature. People are busier than ever, so they inevitably turn to book reviews, talk shows, and drive-time radio to help become informed about the latest in the health and fitness field. Sadly, sound bites become the primary source of information.

While there *has* been some helpful coverage in newspapers and magazines, and on the Internet and TV, there are also many instances in which a self-proclaimed fitness guru (with limited-to-no experience and/or questionable-to-no credentials) wreaks havoc with people's already confused perceptions.

In other cases, so-called fitness experts have seemingly impressive credentials, such as Ph.D., M.D. or R.D., which people have been taught to trust. Unless,
however, their degree is in an area of exercise science (for example, exercise
physiology, biomechanics, or kinesiology), chances are the degree does not
qualify them to write or speak about fitness.

The first step in myth-busting is to arm yourself with knowledge. The more
knowledge you have, the more resistant you are to false claims, false prophets,
and falsehoods.

To minimize being misled by these falsehoods taught by non-professionals,
be mindful of the source from which the information is derived. There are academic and professional credentials specific to the exercise sciences, and college programs teach various aspects of fitness, such as biomechanics, exercise
physiology, or kinesiology, at all levels of higher education (undergraduate,
graduate, and doctorate).

Certifications require a broad basic understanding of how the human body
functions. Some of the more reputable certifying associations are: the American College of Sports Medicine (ACSM), and the American Council on Exercise
(ACE), and the National Strength and Conditioning Association (NSCA), and
each of these organizations have continuing education requirements that must
be satisfied every two years in order to maintain certification.

In summary, avoid believing everything you see on TV, or read in newspapers, magazines, and the Internet. While these sources do sometimes have reputable information, seeking it out is akin to separating wheat from chaff.

Try to find information that offers a variety of scientific references supporting what is being taught. As you delve more closely into those periodicals con-
taining more fact than fiction, take note of the professional publications that
consistently contain quality information. Stick with them. Exercise is, after all, a
science (as well as an art). And every science requires some amount of research.

In the meantime, allow me to introduce you to the contemporary world's
most common, destructive, and mythical fitness ideas.

On Environment

Myth 1

We have little or no control over health and aging,
which are solely determined by genetics.

Truth. While genetics is a contributing factor, lifestyle choices are the single largest factors influencing how healthy you are and how you age. Blaming your genes is a self-defeating excuse that simply perpetuates the myth. If genetics was the sole precursor to wellness, then the genes of our predecessors (from the pre-fast food, TV, and computerization eras) should have safeguarded everyone. You do not have to be a geneticist to see the reality of the matter.

By comparing graduation photos of elementary, high school, or college students from the 1940s and '50s with photos of students from today's classes, it becomes apparent that the genetics of the older generations were not strong enough to keep subsequent generations from getting heavier.

Today, in fact, more than 66 percent of American adults are overweight (as compared with 20 percent in the 1950s). If genetics was the main culprit, that should have been enough of a factor in preventing overweight problems in the first place. Clearly, lifestyle choices of inactivity and poor diet have been stronger variables than genetics.

An additional example which disproves the blame-it-all-on-genetics excuse can be seen by comparing populations on a global scale. Let's compare Western culture with Asians, who are known to be slimmer. Obesity rates are much lower in China and Japan than in America's Chinese and Japanese populations. If genetics is the primary reason for overweight, Asians should be slim regardless of where they live. The same is true for Italians. Those living in Italy tend to be slimmer than Italian-Americans. Apparently, the genes of Italians who emigrated to America didn't protect their offspring from becoming more overweight than the Italians back in Italy.

Such comparisons can also be applied to a variety of health issues, ranging from cancer to diabetes. In the industrialized world, Japanese women have one of the lowest rates of breast cancer, while women in America have one of the highest rates. After just one generation in the United States, however, women of Japanese descent end up with breast cancer rates equal to the overall average for American women. Imagine that—Japan is a culture with 2,000 years of history, and yet that is not enough to protect its people from the deleterious effects of an American lifestyle. One generation of American lifestyle is all it took to erase a long history of health and longer life.

Myth 2

Most diseases are uncontrollable since environmental toxins cause them.

Truth. Those who claim the problem is environmental (air and water pollution) are overlooking the fact that, in some ways, Japan is more environmentally toxic than the United States. If you include New Zealand in the comparison, it would become apparent that environmental pollution is not as big a factor as diet and exercise.

New Zealand is a more agrarian culture than either the United States or Japan. Yet, New Zealand's rates of colon cancer are similar to the United States, while Japan's rate is much lower. New Zealand's environment is markedly different from America's, but their lifestyle of poor diet and lack of activity are similar. Lifestyle choices, such as quality of nutrients consumed, physical-activity levels, and sleep patterns, that are made on a day-to-day basis are paramount to health and longevity.

On Exercise

Myth 3

Strength training is only for young people.

Truth. Strength training is beneficial for people of *all* ages. Why discriminate against age? This is merely an excuse for those who just don't want to move their gluteals (buttocks). If anyone needs to exercise more, it is older people, who, after all, tend to be more sedentary in their daily existence.

I'll never forget the time the manager of a restaurant I frequented asked me why I continued to exercise so intensely. He mentioned that there was no longer a purpose for exercise, for either of us, since both of us had already reached the *ripe old age* of . . . thirty-two. Stunned by the shallowness of his reasoning, I froze momentarily, unable to offer the list of endless benefits that can result from this wonderfully powerful activity.

What he was probably referring to was the purely superficial perspective of appearance. Perhaps he felt that, at thirty-two, few people could look the way they did when they were eighteen. I disagree. Some people can, in fact, look even better.

Even if what he was saying was true, however, I wondered how anyone could possibly *not* care about how they look at *any* point in life. Why, I wondered, should anyone give up on looking good? I recall how my grandmother fussed to look good just to answer the door when a package was delivered—and she was ninety-two at the time. But over and above that argument, I now know that exercise transcends mere concerns with appearance. It is more than just a shallow luxury; it is essential for a fully functioning life, particularly as people age.

An Olympic marathon runner once said, "You don't stop exercising because you grow old. You grow old because you stop exercising." Numerous studies have shown that formerly sedentary older people experienced dramatic positive changes from steady, intense exercise programs for periods as short as twelve weeks.

Myth 4

Strength training is only for building a bulky physique.

Truth. Weight training is merely a tool. How that tool is used is what determines the eventual outcome. (I must admit, however, that I, too, held onto this myth for many years. Although I was active through my college years, I felt there was no need for anything as formal and rigorous as strength training. My fear was that if I lifted weights, I'd look like a gorilla within two weeks.)

There are several variables that can be manipulated to attain the results you are seeking: The amount of resistance; the number of reps and sets; and the rest intervals between the sets, exercises, and workouts. Anyone can design a routine to produce the results he or she chooses, whether the goal is to build up, trim down, or even recover from disease or injury. In light of the lifestyle of convenience people have evolved into, it is necessary for everyone—young and old, male and female—to challenge their bodies with the irreplaceable modality of exercise.

Myth 5

Strength training is only good for men.

Truth. Strength training is equally important for both sexes. It is so good to see more and more women getting interested in strength training. Yet, unfortunately, many others still shy away from this vital part of a well-rounded physical regime because, when it comes to strength training, the primary concern for most women is that they will build masculine bodies.

It saddens and frustrates me when a woman tells me she fears any form of strength training, believing it will make her look like Arnold Schwarzenegger's twin sister even if only light resistance is applied. First of all, it takes years of dedicated effort to build huge muscles. Secondly, a woman would need the testosterone levels of a man in order to develop muscles like a man. Or, she would have to use steroids and male growth hormones—a very sick approach to striving for strength increases or improvements in shape. This is one of those cases where a little information goes a long way, but a little *mis*-information goes a lot further.

In the highly unlikely event that a woman happens to generate more muscle tissue than intended, she need only stop training as intensely. Within five to seven days, muscle tissue will begin to atrophy (although the real solution would be to modify the variables involved in a strength-training program, as discussed in Chapter 9).

In some respects, strength training may be very important for women, particularly for the prevention or management of diminished bone density due to osteoporosis. Inasmuch as women are more susceptible to osteoporosis than men, it is critical that they consider strength training, which, among many other benefits, increases bone density. Also, the increased muscle density resulting from strength training will permanently elevate metabolism and contribute to more efficient fat-burning, a major concern for most women.

Myth 6

After being on a strength-training program,
muscles will turn to fat if the program is halted.

Truth. This is virtually impossible, because muscles and fat are two entirely different forms of tissue. One cannot be converted into the other. It's the same as comparing apples and oranges.

If you cease training, you *will* lose muscle tissue. Consequently, there will be a decrease in metabolism and an eventual increase in fat tissue—probably the fat you would already have accumulated had you not strength trained at all.

Myth 7

To trim your waistline, do more crunches.

Truth. Unfortunately, there is no such thing as spot-reducing fat. You can *spot-train* muscles—or, in other words, train specific muscles in an isolated fashion (which, in essence, is what crunches do—they spot-train your abdominals).

However, fat-burning is a more complex process and results from a variety of factors, not just one specific exercise. One is to increase muscle tissue through strength training. Another is to incorporate cardiovascular conditioning, which involves performing aerobic exercises for a minimum of twenty minutes, four to six times a week.

A third factor contributing to a trimmer waistline comes via your mouth in the form of proper nutrition (see Myth 8 below). This means two things: First, you must maintain the appropriate balance between calories consumed and calories expended (through physical activities and exercise), and second, it is critical to be mindful of the *quality* of calories consumed. For instance, it should come as no surprise to you that 500 calories consumed from a bowl of Neapolitan ice cream is less healthy for you than 500 calories consumed from a bowl of homemade chicken soup.

On Diet

Myth 8

A high-protein, low-carbohydrate diet is best for getting into shape.

Truth. In order to get into better shape, exercise is essential. In order to have the energy to exercise with the intensity needed for optimal results, proper nourishment becomes a priority. The best source for energy is carbohydrates—specifically, complex carbohydrates with a low-glycemic value (see Chapter 5). These carbohydrates, which are digested more slowly, cause a minimal rise in insulin, are not converted to fat very easily, and provide more energy than simple carbohydrates). Examples include brown rice, vegetables, and wholegrain breads and cereals. In addition to fueling muscles, carbohydrates are the sole source of fuel for the brain.

The media had a field day glorifying the high-protein diet—you only heard the success stories (though what is defined as a so-called success is questionable—it's not just about weight loss). Having worked, and worked out, on the gym floors of the fitness industry day in and day out for twenty plus years, I've heard the good, the bad, and the ugly on this particular topic.

From locker room discussions to talk on the gym floor, it seems that for each person who felt good while on this diet, there were at least ten others who felt absolutely awful. Some of my many gym acquaintances actually saw their exercise performance decline while consuming few carbohydrates. If I lived on the high-protein diet, I know full well I wouldn't have the energy to do the work I do, twelve to fourteen hours a day, running from gym to home office to the next gym and back. In fact, every week, people comment on how I always seem to be so full of energy—always running around, full of zest. I attribute that to my high intake of complex carbohydrates. It's certainly not due to rest, which I usually lack (although I am working on improving this critical element).

The primary purpose of protein is for the growth and repair of body tissues. Since the body already manufactures its own protein (with the exception of nine essential amino acids), excess protein places stress on the kidneys and liver. When too few carbohydrates are consumed, the body becomes dehydrated, thereby causing a host of problems resulting from the respective losses in minerals.

Protein sources boost the metabolism more than carbohydrates and require more time to be digested and assimilated. Consuming protein prior to a workout would, therefore, cause muscle fatigue more readily. Conversely, complex carbohydrates provide the fuel needed by the muscles for work. Weight training is essential for the strengthening of muscle tissue and for the permanent elevation of metabolism. In order to work out with greater energy and intensity, complex carbohydrates—the most efficient fuel—must be consumed prior to working out.

Bottom line: Don't buy into the hype. Today's fad diet books, whether about low, no, or all carbohydrates—are destined for the clearance bin by next diet-book season. It's important to have a proper balance of all three *macronutrients* (carbohydrates, fats, and proteins), the primary nutrients responsible for the maintenance of bodily functions at rest and during physical activity. (See Chapter 5 for more on macronutrients.)

Myth 9

There are no bad foods.

Truth. Many authors and dietitians claim that, with moderation, *all* foods can be included in the diet. This is a dangerous perspective because there are many foods that can more easily contribute to excess fat and a number of other serious health problems. Don't get me wrong, I do believe in cheating by treating yourself to junk food *occasionally.* However, incorporating toxic foods (hot dogs, French fries, bacon, etc.) on even an occasional basis is counterproductive to health and fitness. Eating the wrong types of foods can easily lead to problems, such as colon cancer, diabetes, obesity, and osteoporosis.

Myth 10

To lose weight, eat only one or two meals per day.

Truth. Eating too few meals will actually slow down your metabolism and lead to cumulative increases in fat over time. In fact, even the traditional three-square-meals approach is unhealthy. It is important to eat a minimum of four times a day, with a goal of five or six times a day. To burn fat, you need to eat more frequently. It has become obvious to me, as a trainer interacting with hundreds of people every week, that the leanest, shapeliest, most-toned people are those who eat four or more times a day. In fact, people who have higher body-fat levels tend to skip meals or eat only twice a day.

As discussed in Chapter 5, metabolism stays elevated with frequent eating, but drops precipitously when too many hours lapse between meals. Unfortunately, many of the uninitiated will take this news and run with it, eating not only more often, but just plain eating *more*. The key here is to eat *fewer calories* at each meal. Just by eating the same daily number of calories over more meals, your metabolism should improve.

Myth 11

If you eat a well-balanced diet, there should be no need for supplements.

Truth. With all the existing environmental issues, such as depleted topsoil, pesticide and herbicide usage, polluted air, and toxic waters, it is not possible to have a well-balanced diet in the purest sense of the word. Too many micronutrients and elements have been diminished, if not eliminated, for foods to contain the nourishment they were meant to provide. While the media has focused on herbs and supplements that have medicinal properties (and, therefore, potentially negative side effects), there are many others that are food-grade (non-toxic), and provide only positive results. To understand what is best for your individual needs, it would be a great idea to either speak with a knowledgeable person in a health food store, a family doctor trained in nutrition, or consult with a nutritionist, if possible.

Myth 12

To prevent unwanted weight gain, avoid eating after 7:00 PM

Truth. There is no such exact formula. The timing of your last meal should be based on what time you go to sleep as well as the level of activity that will be performed after the meal is completed. It takes the body approximately three to four hours to digest the food of an average-sized meal. If you typically go to bed at 1:00 AM, then too many hours will pass between 7:00 PM and bedtime, thereby contributing to a slower metabolism. Due to my work schedule (I am usually at the gym until 11:30 PM), I generally don't get to sleep until 4:00 AM. If I stopped eating at 7:00 PM, I'd be wreaking havoc on my metabolism, as well as my blood sugar.

On General Health

Myth 13

To measure progress, weigh yourself on a scale regularly.

Truth. The scale is perhaps the most misleading gauge for fitness progress. When you weigh yourself, do you know how much of that weight is fat and how much is lean tissue? Of course you don't. The number you see on the scale is a measure of everything you are made of—this includes bones, brains, fat, muscles, organs, and skin.

When I first joined a gym at the age of twenty-three, I exercised diligently and ate healthfully. As the weeks passed, I started to feel trimmer and tighter around the waist, firmer and stronger overall due to my increased muscle tone. Sensing I was lighter on my feet after twelve weeks of this new lifestyle, I decided to weigh myself, believing I should have lost at least several pounds by then. To my surprise (and confusion), not only had I *not* lost any weight, I had actually gained five pounds. That was my first lesson in understanding that muscles weigh much more than fat and that the scale can be misleading in determining success.

When people go on fad diets, such as starvation or high-protein/low-carbohydrate diets, the body *does* shed pounds, but not fat weight. The first pounds to be shed with any extreme diet approach are usually water and muscle weight. Since muscle tissue dictates how high metabolic rates are, the loss of muscle will lead to higher fat levels. Consequently, although you may appear lighter according to the scale, you may actually be fatter and, thus, less healthy. The resulting elevated body-fat percentage will create a higher susceptibility to a variety of diseases.

So how can you gauge progress? You can have your body-fat percentage estimated and tape measurements recorded (as discussed in Chapter 6), or you can, more simply, judge by how your clothing fits. What comes to mind is how my grandfather always bragged that his weight at the age of seventy was the same as it had been forty-five years earlier. What he failed to realize was that what used to be a V-shape had become an upside-down V-shape, with his waistline slowly increasing from twenty-nine to a measurement of forty-one. I'm afraid to imagine his shift in body-fat percentages.

Myth 14

People who work out are narcissistic.

Truth. Although subjective and not directly supported by research studies, this is not typically the case. Granted, there are people who exercise simply to impress others with a nice body. However, many who stay with a workout routine long enough recognize the healing power of such activities. They transcend the desire for mere aesthetic improvements and move on to appreciating the mental, physical, and spiritual health benefits associated with exercise. By attaining a heightened level of physical and mental awareness, people are better able to manage their emotions and tap into their spiritual awareness. In addition to finding it easier to live with people who are at peace with themselves, it should also be comforting to know they will more easily maintain independent lifestyles than would be the case if they did not exercise.

True narcissism is when people, in an attempt to relax or feel good, abuse alcohol and/or drugs and smoke cigarettes or cigars. In each of these cases, they are not just hurting themselves, but those around them.

Myth 15

Excess body weight is fine since it is merely an aesthetic choice.

Truth. Attempting to remain slim or reduce fat is more than just an issue of appearance. Numerous studies have illustrated the deleterious effects of excess fat on health and longevity. According to a study published in the *International Journal of Cancer,* excess fat has been linked to cancer in several parts of the body, including the breast, colon, gallbladder, and prostate.

Sal's Summary

There are numerous myths and misconceptions that can sabotage any earnest effort to achieve a healthier existence. Although the above myths are merely a sampling of erroneous misconceptions, understanding them will help you develop an ability to decipher truth from falsehood (if in doubt, feel free to visit the websites listed in the Resources section in back).

I have been blessed with a mother who has always lived her life free of any limiting thoughts about aging and she was always a positive role model for me. At times, I lost sight of her age, often thinking of her more as an older sister. Her sense of humor, her agility, and her athleticism made me view her as just one of the other kids. Whenever I met the parents of friends, I felt as though they were my mom's elders, not realizing they were either the same age, or perhaps even younger than she was.

In some ways, I became spoiled, maintaining high expectations of other older people. But it didn't occur to me until my late teens and early twenties that my mom's peers appeared much older because they chose to act the way adults are supposed to act—with slower, refined (old-age) movements. They weren't supposed to roller skate, bike ride along the bike paths, or play basketball or handball in the parks. Running for a Frisbee, or simply wrestling for the heck of it was totally out of the question—but these are the very activities that keep people young.

Older adults simply need to remember how to play like kids again. And if you've been sedentary for too long to return to such activities right now, then condition yourself, slowly but surely, to at least begin participating in a few. Some other ideas for activities include power walking, swimming, tennis, and even dancing, whether it is square dancing, swing, or Latin dancing . . . as long as it is fast dancing.

Whatever you do, try your best to avoid the standard roll-over-and-play-dead lifestyle. The human body was designed to be in motion. Just as in Newton's law, "an object in motion tends to stay in motion—an object at rest tends to stay at rest." In layman's terms: The more you stay seated, the more you'll need to sit.

As you become more sedentary (a *choice*), your circulation of blood, oxygen, and nutrients begin to slow down. And, as this occurs, your ligaments, muscles, and tendons begin to shorten and lose flexibility and strength.

If you sit at a desk job all day, be sure to take a long, brisk walk at lunchtime. Not permitted to take lunch breaks? Then change jobs. If finding a new job is unrealistic, then get up periodically and walk around—to the water fountain, the rest room, the lobby for a pack of tissues. Whatever you choose, just create reasons to move your body, and your body will reward you with a more youthful existence.

2

What Happens As You Age

For starters, I want to address one basic, seemingly easy question: What, exactly, *is* aging? Many times, when I start a program with a new client, they establish pre-existing limitations on themselves based on their age—not their individual capabilities. When I suggest higher levels of activity with increased intensity, the same answer comes back to me time and time again: "Do you know how *old* I am?" I've heard that phrase so many times, I can practically say it along with them. My best answer to that is to ask if *they* know what their age is.

Without overanalyzing, stop reading for sixty seconds and allow your thoughts and feelings about aging to surface fully. Does your first impression involve a number? If so, then you're relying on the less accurate measure of *chronological* aging. When you hear the word aging, do you envision yourself as fat, or frail? Or how about being unable to move around without assistance?

These images are typically conjured up with the word aging. Yet there is so much more to aging than simply counting the number of years lived, though only a small minority may actually envision themselves doing exactly what they have always enjoyed doing, regardless of age.

Another type of aging to be aware of—which is more accurate as a gauge—is *biological* aging. From as early as my high school years, I've had numerous acquaintances who would prefer living shorter lives simply to avoid that dreaded old age. Hearing this has always perplexed me, since I have always had a different perception of what being old means, mainly because I was fortunate enough to be raised by parents who set unspoken examples about aging, or more appropriately, the lack thereof.

My mom, who has always been active, continues to exercise and play sports to this day, while my dad continues to watch TV. The problem for my dad, however, is that if he tries to exert himself much beyond the activity of walking from his TV chair to the kitchen or bathroom, he begins to feel aches and tightness that encourage him to remain seated.

Many will recognize this self-fulfilling prophecy. This is why many exercise machines become little more than clothes hangers or extended closets a week or two after they've been delivered and get used once, twice, or maybe three times. What happens is, their owners get sore each time because it's been so long between acts of physical exertion, and from then on, the machines become naturally associated with pain. Thus the rows of clothes hangers taking up space where biceps or abdominals should still be exercised.

My mom, however, bowls in four leagues, lifts weights two to three times per week, plays handball twice a week, and regularly takes brisk one-hour walks. Although my dad likes to attribute her higher strength and energy levels to the fact that she is younger than him, a four-year age difference is insignificant when compared to her level of regular activity. And, at seventy-five years, my mom is not exactly a spring chicken. (Incidentally, the being-younger excuse has been used by my dad for over thirty years, from the time they were both in their forties.)

This chapter presents the bad news and the good news about aging—first the warning, then the inspiration to take action. The bad news is not intended to depress you, but instead make you aware of the degenerative processes generally associated with aging. In knowing about degeneration, you will be more impressed with the good news—your body's ability to regenerate through proper diet and exercise.

First, The Bad News

Physiology, or the ability to perform activities, improves most rapidly during childhood and peaks sometime between the late teenage years and the thirties. By the fourth decade, the body begins to degenerate more rapidly than it can be regenerated, causing many simultaneous changes. Overall muscle mass and strength decline by 30–50 percent between the ages of thirty and eighty, with associated reductions in bone density. Particularly after the age of forty, people start losing one quarter to one third of a pound of muscle tissue each year. Although this may seem insignificant, such losses lead to a one- to two-percent reduction in strength each year. This results in a steady decline in metabolism and a steady increase in fat accumulation. With these developments comes an increased risk for diseases, such as cancer, diabetes, hypertension, and osteoporosis.

Sedentary living equates to reductions in the amount of the much-needed physical stress we should be placing on our bodies. Functional capabilities (the ability to perform everyday tasks) begin to diminish over time. Movements become slower as reaction time, coordination, and balance decline, increasing the risk of falls. As a result of lowered bone mass, such falls, however minor, can be crippling—even fatal.

Other degenerative symptoms include atherosclerosis (the formation and accumulation of plaques—cholesterol-rich deposits—in arteries), depression, increases in blood pressure and cholesterol, a reduction in aerobic capacity, slower mental functioning, and a weakened immune system overall. All these factors are interrelated—the degeneration of one element contributes to the degeneration of another.

Muscle loss is the catalyst that sparks the overall downward spiral erroneously blamed on aging. Muscle tissue is linked with balance, gait, and strength. Decreases in muscle tissue are directly associated with increases in difficulty functioning on a day-to-day basis—carrying groceries, doing laundry, going up and down stairs, opening bottles of water or jars of food, and even rising from a chair becomes difficult, if not impossible. The relationship between muscular strength and quality of life is extremely important, and there is much that can be done to slow down, even reverse, the age-related degeneration of muscle tissue.

Are you depressed yet? If so, then it's time for you to take action. The first step is by learning the good news. And, believe me, there is plenty.

Now, the Good News

The good news is that this supposedly inevitable degeneration can, in fact, be minimized, slowed down, and even averted. It is so exciting that you *do* have the choice to either degenerate quickly or live youthfully all your life. Although previously deemed as simply out of your control, declines such as muscle atrophy and diminished cardiovascular capacity are now known to be caused by sedentary lifestyles more than aging. The rest of this book teaches methods that can make the slowdown, even reversal, of aging possible.

In order to see how it is possible to slow down or stop aging, it is vital to first understand the different types of aging. The most widely recognized is *chronological age*. This relates to the amount of time a person has lived, expressed by the number of years and months since birth. The type of aging described earlier in this chapter is most readily associated with this category. The problem with referring to chronological age as a gauge is that it does not take into consideration biological, psychological, or sociological factors.

Getting older is an inevitable fact of life. It is a universal phenomenon everyone experiences. But time is a limited measure, calculated in a simple, linear pattern. It is also relative: What may be deemed old age in American culture may be considered only middle age in another culture. The question should not be how many years you have accumulated, or how old you are, but rather, how quickly aging has occurred independent of time.

To fully understand the true meaning of aging, it is critical to recognize measures of the aging process that help compare differences for people of the same chronological age. Such measures fall under the category of *functional age,* and included in this category are biological age, psychological age, and social age.

There was a *Twilight Zone* episode that had strong parallels to what is being taught here about aging. Although I saw it only once, when I was in my early teens, it left a lasting impression. Some of you may remember it.

The story was about the residents of an old-age home in a suburban town. One of the residents cheerfully tried to recruit as many of the other residents as possible to play a game of Kick the Can. At first, he was only able to convince a few of his peers. But as time passed, more and more joined in for what turned out to be laugh-filled, childlike games. The fun was contagious. Throughout the story, however, there was one irritable resident who opposed the thought of "being absurd and immature." He viewed the main character as a quack and tried to discourage everyone else from playing, out of fear of creating injuries or breaking the rules. He refused, he said, to "act like a child."

In the final scene, all the residents except this grumpy man agreed to play a game out on the lawn at night. From inside the home, the lone resident could hear his housemates laughing with joy as the game got underway. As the game progressed, he suddenly became aware that the voices outside were those of youngsters—not old adults. Going out on the porch, he was astonished to see a group of children running on the lawn. As he called out to them, they all dispersed, running and laughing into the darkness of the night, leaving him to age all by himself. In true *Twilight Zone* fashion, through their youthful activity and mindsets, the residents of this retirement home were literally able to regain their youth.

While it is, of course, impossible to reverse the hands of time, as happened in this memorable story, it *is* possible to reverse its effects. The moral here is simple: Play, keep active, and forever feel the joy of movement. While doing this won't literally turn you into a kid again, it will allow you to escape, or at least minimize, the effects of old age . . . not in terms of chronological age, as with the show, but in terms of physiological, psychological, and sociological factors. With all these positive benefits, why focus on a silly, redundant number referred to as *age*?

Instead, it's time to turn to the positive and see how to reverse that number.

Why Strength Training Increases Youthfulness

All the degenerative effects of aging can be referred to as typical changes, to be distinguished from what may be categorized as *necessary* changes. *Necessary* changes are those which, by the laws of human nature, are inevitable, regardless of what you do or how you live your life. *Typical* changes are those occuring due to customary, day-to-day lifestyle choices. The purpose of this chapter is to show you how you can avoid, eliminate, or reverse the *typical* changes associated with aging—or, more accurately, sedentary living (diminished muscular strength, diminished bone density, weakened joints, and slower, weaker movements, to name a few).

The tendency (translation: the *choice*) to become increasingly less active is the critical element that has long been overlooked by studies examining the effects of aging. Activities that tend to become minimized or eliminated are the very ones that are most essential for keeping bodies stronger and younger. As people age, they tend to avoid activities which require brisk movement for extended periods of time (long brisk walks or jogs, bicycle rides, etc.), or activities that challenge their muscles and bones (lifting and carrying heavy objects, such as groceries, book bags, etc.).

Regardless of what sports you play and/or what style of exercise you prefer, whether it's aerobics, Pilates, tai chi, yoga, or any other form, strength training is at the very core of preparing you for a more active, fruitful, *younger* lifestyle. (See "Sports Do Not Replace Exercise" on page 29.) It is an integral part of any and every form of physical activity. I'm not suggesting that it replace other exercise methods. Instead, I'm merely suggesting that no other method replaces strength training. All styles of exercise are beneficial in a variety of ways. One isn't better than the other, and, in many ways, they are complementary.

The most popular modes of exercise that are helpful in maintaining a more healthful and youthful existence include a variety of options, each with several overlapping benefits, as well as benefits specific to their own method. These are: Balance, cardiovascular, flexibility, and strength training. Of Far-Eastern origin, there is tai-chi chuan, qigong, and yoga. And then there are such Western-derived methods as Feldenkrais, Pilates, and The Alexander technique.

Although each style is beneficial for the human body, strength training—a long overlooked approach to wellness—is truly the foundation for all forms of exercise, sports, and overall basic human activity, such as climbing, lifting, and walking. It is the primary way that age-related declines in strength and muscle mass can be most easily halted or reversed.

Numerous studies have demonstrated that even up to 100 years of age, men and women maintain their ability to increase muscle strength. Even if increases in muscular strength were the sole benefit derived from strength training, it would be enough of an impact to dramatically improve the quality and quantity of life.

Until recently, the healing powers of strength training had been widely misunderstood and grossly underestimated. As exercise became increasingly popular in the 1960s and '70s, working out aerobically was touted as *the* exercise solution for wellness. Now it appears that yoga and tai chi have moved into the limelight. Granted, aerobics and yoga—and all the others—are essential for the

SPORTS DO NOT REPLACE EXERCISE

Sports and exercise are two entirely different classifications of activities. Too many times, when I asked acquaintances whether they worked out, they would answer, "Yes, I play basketball (or tennis)." What they didn't realize is that sports challenge the integrity of the joints and break down muscle fibers. On the other hand, working out through strength conditioning prepares the body for sport. While both activity styles burn calories and challenge the body physically, each offers different benefits. Avoid the misconception that playing basketball, tennis, or any other sport, replaces a well-designed workout . . . they are two entirely different entities.

benefits that are specific to those forms of exercise, such as flexibility and improved breathing patterns. But, unless you strengthen muscles through strength-training exercises, you will not be able to perform at the same level of intensity and endurance.

Incidentally, due to the repetitive nature of aerobic exercise, yoga, and most sports, there is potential risk for muscle tears and joint strain due to overuse. In order to strengthen a joint, you must strengthen the muscles surrounding that joint. Through strength training, the potential for injury is minimized. Tendons and ligaments (connective tissue for muscles and bones), which are vulnerable to the stresses of many activities, become stronger. Also, the bones, to which the tendons are attached, become thicker.

The Confusion Between Muscular Endurance and Muscular Strength

There is a world of difference between muscular endurance and muscular strength. Increases in strength will enhance endurance, but muscular endurance will not enhance muscular strength. While exercise modalities, such as aerobics, calisthenics (chin-ups, pushups, and sit-ups), Pilates, and yoga all enhance muscular endurance, they do little for muscular strength. The exception, of course, is for beginners and formerly sedentary people. In these cases, any form of activity provides enough shock to the body to elicit strength gains. (See Chapter 9 for a detailed description of the elements needed for strength increases.)

However, with calisthenics or yoga, as a person becomes stronger, the only way to continually challenge the body is by increasing the number of repetitions or the amount of time poses are held. By doing increasing numbers of chin-ups, pushups, and sit-ups, or by holding poses for longer and longer periods of time, muscles are not being challenged in a way that will elicit strength increases, but will rather enhance endurance only. Simply put, nothing strengthens muscles, bones, and connective tissue (ligaments and tendons) the way that strength training does. Nothing can replace strength training for many of the benefits it offers.

The Many Benefits of Strength Training

There is endless, compelling evidence supporting the need for strength training for all populations, from early teens to senior citizens. It is absolutely remark-

able how something as seemingly crude as strength training can be so powerfully beneficial in a variety of ways, for all humans, of all ages. It is exciting to
know that such a basic form of exercise can do so much to improve your quality of life, help prevent diseases—or manage existing ones—and sculpt the
body in the exact way you choose (within the scope of your body type).

Many years ago, and even today in some circles, strength training was
viewed solely as a tool for building huge muscles and developing bulky
physiques, with a consequential loss of flexibility and functionality. It was also
perceived that if a person had high blood pressure and/or needed to lose
weight, it was best to avoid strength-training exercises, and primarily perform
aerobic exercises.

Many people, including sports coaches and athletic trainers, frowned upon
this powerful method of exercise. They suspected that training with resistance
would interfere with sports performance. In fact, when I was on a track team in
high school during the early 1970s, my coach prohibited our team from lifting
weights, particularly for the lower body, out of fear of getting too bulky and losing speed and flexibility. How mistaken everyone was. Not only are athletes of
all types (strength or speed) strength training, but so are ballet dancers and
even people with cancer, heart disease, and injuries.

It has become evident that muscle tissue actually burns fat, and perhaps
more efficiently with strength training than by doing aerobics, swimming,
yoga, or just about any other form of exercise. (See "How Swimming Compares
with Strength Training" on page 33.) Excess fat is deadly on so many levels—it
serves as a storage site for carcinogens, and it creates imbalances in hormonal
levels, thereby allowing for a host of hormone-related diseases (cancer of the
breast, cervix, liver, ovary, pancreas, and prostate, to name a few).

As is now known, strength training is vastly more beneficial and sophisti-
cated than it was previously perceived to be. Its recognized benefits are numerous, and they continue to increase in variety. To help you recognize the power
and beauty of strength training, here is a list of fifteen potential benefits associated with it.

1. It lowers LDL (bad) cholesterol and elevates HDL (good) cholesterol. Studies have shown that as little as five months of strength training resulted in
   significant decreases in total cholesterol and LDL cholesterol.

2. It can prevent or help regulate diabetes. Strength training is effective in
   improving insulin sensitivity and glucose tolerance.

3. It strengthens your heart due to increased thickness in the wall of the heart. Just as with any muscle in your skeletal system, the heart muscle becomes stronger through strength training. This helps the heart function more efficiently, allowing for less stress and less pressure to be placed on it. Strength training is so beneficial for the heart, it is commonly used as part of cardiac rehabilitation programs for people with heart disease.

4. It reduces blood pressure and heart rate. This is due to the strengthening of the heart, which, in turn, helps it to function more efficiently. Another variable is that artery stiffening (commonly associated with aging), a condition that causes increases in blood pressure, is reduced.

5. It increases muscle tissue and strength. Without added outside resistance, muscles atrophy (disintegrate). To become strong and to stay strong, muscles need to be stimulated with more resistance than they have grown accustomed to (adaptation). One primary advantage of strength training is the ability to apply *overload* (applying a greater level of intensity than the muscles are accustomed to).

6. It strengthens ligaments and tendons (connective tissue). Strength training doesn't only strengthen muscle tissue. It also affects everything that muscle is attached to—muscles attach to bones via tendons, bones attach to bones via ligaments.

7. It thickens bone density, minimizing the chances for osteoporosis (for the same reason as #6 above).

8. It reduces pain and improves function for those with arthritis. Stronger muscles lessen the stress on joints by absorbing the shock caused by everyday activities.

9. It elevates continuous round-the-clock metabolism, thereby permanently reducing fat storage. Muscles require more energy (calories) to be maintained.

10. It increases *muscular endurance,* therefore increasing the ability to develop aerobic endurance. The stronger a muscle is, the longer it takes for that muscle to fatigue.

11. It improves mental clarity and the sense of well-being, thereby reducing levels of depression. Mental functioning benefits due to improvements in blood flow throughout the body, including the brain. With increased strength comes an increased number of activities that can be performed,

resulting in an elevated sense of satisfaction with life and an improved perception of the self. Also, strength training increases the feel-good hormones. Some examples include adrenalin, endorphins, and testosterone (which help people feel stronger and more energized).

12. It enhances flexibility when exercising with the proper range of motion (ROM). (Flexibility is defined as the ROM at a joint.) The stronger a joint is, the better it can function through its ROM.

13. It enhances mobility and functionality. Strength is needed for daily functioning of basic tasks and for a better quality of life. Through strength training, increases in muscular strength have resulted in improved walking speed, endurance, and mechanics. It has also resulted in improved stair-climbing power. It is essential in helping to prevent falls and disability.

14. It reduces the risk of cancer. Strength training produced favorable changes in several risk factors for cancer—body-fat composition, fasting glucose and insulin, insulinlike growth factors, and waist circumference, to name a few.

15. It minimizes the chances for heart disease. All the major causes for heart disease, such as artery-stiffening, high blood pressure, and high cholesterol, have been shown to be reduced by strength training.

HOW SWIMMING COMPARES WITH STRENGTH TRAINING

There used to be a commonly misunderstood concept that swimming was the best single form of exercise. While it certainly is good exercise, swimming is not even comparable to strength training in terms of the variety of benefits. People tend to be confused about this since, for so many years, they've been told that swimming uses all the muscles of the body. First of all, the resistance provided by water never changes. Muscles, therefore, will adapt to the resistance once the body becomes familiar with the activity, and the strength increases will consequently be minimal. Secondly, swimmers have higher fat content than other athletes—fat is needed for buoyancy and thermal regulation. Lastly, due to the buoyancy of water, swimming is a low-impact activity, which means that little challenge is applied to the skeletal system. This translates to very little benefit for bone health.

A major bonus to all these benefits is that your appearance will improve noticeably. With strength training, you can spot-train specific problem areas or target weaker muscles to help restore muscular balance. When done properly, strength training can help people look, feel, and live as though they are decades younger.

Now, tell me the truth, isn't this stuff exciting? What a beautiful miracle the human body is when it is challenged in the right ways. All these benefits are possible for each and every person, but how many are attainable, and to what extent, depends on you and the effort you choose to apply. Exercise, such as strength training, is merely a tool. How you use the tool is what determines the outcome. *Variety, proper technique,* and *intensity* are the pillars (see Chapter 9), the key variables that can help you live as though you were twenty years younger.

4

Creating Your Plan of Action

B ecoming fitter, healthier, and younger is like taking an exciting journey to a fantastic destination. Like any trip, it can be rewarding, challenging, exotic, and mysterious, and it can produce results that will actually improve and increase your lifetime. And, like any trip, it requires planning, patience, and persistence to turn your dream trip into reality.

As with any trip, it begins with a destination—and a map to get there . . .

The first step in achieving change of any type—body, mind, or soul—comes in the form of goal-setting (the map you'll use to arrive at your destination). Goal-setting should be nothing new to you—in today's world, setting goals is talked of often and loudly. But talking, as you know, doesn't always lead to listening, or in this case, doing. This chapter discusses how to select your goals and, just as importantly, how to reach them. All of this is designed so you will know—and feel in your heart—what you hope to achieve.

Set Goals

As you probably have already experienced in other areas of your life, setting goals is always crucial for inevitable success. Be it the goal to complete college, get a job, propose to a future spouse, have children, or possibly even retire early (and well), goals are at the heart of life's most triumphant moments. They not only help with setting a direction to pursue, they actually point you in the right direction. Goals are like a destination, a place, or a state of mind and body you'd like to reach.

Without goals, motivation is just that—motivation. Call it what you want—

dream, enthusiasm, incentive, or inspiration—a goal without action is little more than an idea. A good idea, but toothless just the same. Anyone can be inspired from time to time to do more, eat less, read a good book, see a block-buster movie, sleep less, walk more, but without a firm goal in place to make those motivations a reality, they remain just so many items on a to-do list that, quite frankly, never gets done.

Two types of goals—long-term and short-term—need to be established in order to succeed. Long-term goals help you begin to take the action needed to generate results that will become evident over the long term (say, six to twelve months, or more, from the current time). In a sense, long-term goals are the big-picture goals—the ones that will impact your longevity and quality of life. Some examples include the ability to walk *longer* distances without resting, measuring by time (twenty minutes longer) or distance (seven blocks more, or a quarter mile more). Such goals help you recognize the relevance and impor-tance of your short-term goals, and, thereby, more easily adhere to healthful day-to-day choices.

Short-term goals (weekly, monthly, and quarterly), help make the attain-ment of long-term goals more palatable, more easily recognizable. Having short-term goals makes it easier to increase your confidence, self-esteem, and enthusiasm by building on these smaller successes while striving for the bigger successes. For example, a short-term goal may be to walk twenty-five minutes a day, four days a week for the next month. At the end of that period, you would then reset your goals, perhaps bumping up the frequency to five days a week, or the length to thirty minutes a day, and/or the speed to 4.0 miles an hour (walk the same distance in less time), or any combination of these.

A strength goal can be to begin lifting weights twice a week for three weeks. Starting in the fourth week, this can be increased to three times a week. Another example would be to lift a given weight, for a bicep curl (where you flex your arm, bringing your hand close to your shoulder), ten consecutive times. When that goal is satisfied, you will feel more confident about the longer-term goal of increasing your muscle's strength by 15 percent. If all you can do are five abdominal crunches, then being able to perform thirty crunches in three months will encourage you to move forward, heading toward your goal of having stronger, firmer abdominals.

The key to achieving both long- and short-term goals is to be realistic. A long-term goal is not to run a marathon next month, any more than a short-term goal is to run a marathon next week. By using realistic short-term goals to reach equally realistic long-term goals, you build on a solid foundation rather than reach for thin air. By setting realistic goals, short-term or long, you can more easily reach *both*.

Recipe for Success—
Make Goals Clear, Concise, and Attainable

In order to remain motivated in the pursuit of your goals, it is necessary to establish goals from the start that are:

Goals
Write your goals down. Being able to see your goals on paper brings them that much closer to fruition.

- Clear

- Concise

- Attainable

Having general goals, such as feeling better, living more healthfully, or even losing weight, are not good enough. Without more specifics, it is easy to veer off course and not even notice it.

For goals to be clear, create ones that are easy to relate to. In lieu of simply aiming to feel better, examples of ideal goals would be to:

- Have more upper body strength

- Be able to play with your children (or grandchildren) longer

- Climb stairs more easily

As you can see, all three specific goals meet the original goal of feeling better, but by being more specific, they are more readily attainable. For instance, climbing stairs more easily can be quantified by comparing how you felt walking up two flights of stairs last week to how you feel performing the same task this week, next week, or even every week. Of course, your goals don't have to be identical to these. Personalize each goal to fit your lifestyle, personality, and desires. Decide what variables or areas of life are most important to you, such as being more active or increasing your strength.

To be concise, goals should be quantifiable. With the goal of developing more upper body strength, you may include in that goal an increase of 10 percent (if you already have a quantifiable record of how much weight you can lift). For playing with your children longer, mention how much longer you would like to play, whether that translates into twenty minutes or one hour. For climbing stairs, you may want to specify an amount of time or the number of flights. Other examples of concise goals can include increasing your walking distance by twenty minutes (or twenty blocks, if you live in a city), losing one pound of fat per week for eight weeks, or trimming your waistline by three inches.

Goals must also be realistically attainable—nothing will sabotage your success more quickly than setting goals that are simply not realistically attainable. If you are five feet tall, and weigh 200 pounds, avoid having a goal of becoming an underweight, six-foot-tall runway model. Even if you *are* six-feet tall, if you have a thicker frame, then avoid striving for a body frame you can't possibly attain. This includes fitting into a size-two pair of jeans or looking like your favorite celebrity or starlet.

For goals that are based on your physical shape, I can make it easier by introducing you to the three basic body types generally referred to in research circles for body assessment:

- Endomorph—Wider, heavier frame with a tendency toward quicker weight (muscle or fat) gain

- Mesomorph—Leaner, more athletic build, with a moderate frame

- Ectomorph—Narrower, slimmer frame with longer, slimmer limbs

Your body type falls into one of these three categories, or somewhere in between any two of them. This assessment method, referred to as *somatotyping,* will help you determine the general category your body fits into, and will help you set realistic goals (and select appropriate role models).

The figures on page 39 illustrates these three basic body types.

Take Action

Now that your goals have been established, it is important to grasp the philosophy that *it's not just the destination, but the journey that matters.* It is through your journey, after all, that you will grow, not just in terms of physical health, but also spiritually and emotionally.

Practicing healthful lifestyle habits helps to build character. It teaches you about devotion, persistence, diligence, and focus—admirable qualities, which, once cultivated, will be yours forever. When people seek shortcuts, such as diet pills, liposuction, and stomach stapling, they miss out on a fabulous journey of

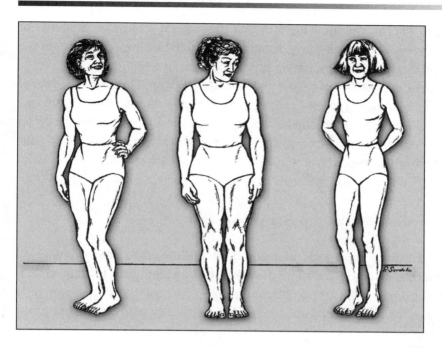

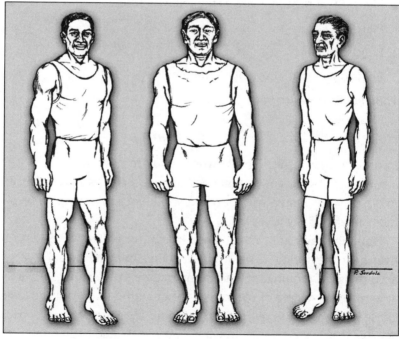

The three basic body types for females (top) and males (bottom).

growth . . . not to mention the fact that they spend enormous amounts of money and risk their well-being, if not their very lives, simply to shortcut the journey and reach their destination just that much quicker.

Of course, every journey begins with a single footstep. This first step, one of many, implies action. Therefore, every journey begins with action, and so, too, will yours. The good thing about stepping into action is that once you're on your journey, every step—every action—brings you closer and closer to your destination. And again, it's on the journey that you learn so much. This is what is meant by the phrase *enjoy the ride.*

P-R-E-P Yourself

After establishing your goals and committing yourself to actively reaching them, there is some degree of prep work that is needed prior to starting with the actual exercises. This is no different from preparing for any other trip, only in this case, the destination is not some beach house or theme park, but a better, happier, healthier, and even longer life.

My PREP approach involves the following steps:

1. **P**lan

2. Be **R**ealistic

3. **E**nvision your attainment of your goals

4. Be **P**ersistent with your actions

Plan

In order to get from point A (where you are now) to point B (the successful attainment of your goals), you need to have a clear and concise plan of action. In other words, you must not only get out your road map (your plan), but you must actually draw it, as well.

Nothing that you have achieved in life—or will achieve—was by accident. Ever hear the saying, *there are no accidents in the universe*? Everything you've accomplished required at least some degree of effort, which was preceded by at least some degree of planning—the attainment of a college degree, the purchase of a car or a house. Even winning the lotto takes a conscious plan to achieve the desired result. To win at lotto, you need to plan three steps: Go to a store, choose a set of numbers, and pay with money you brought for that purpose. So, while winning may feel like chance, it is actually the result of a clear and conscious plan.

Health and fitness is no different. Yet, so many people don't take it seriously enough to recognize that health also requires a set of plans. As the apt cliché goes, *Failing to plan is planning to fail.* Especially with fitness, it is too easy to blow it off the moment something else comes up—a work project, a social obligation, or simply a TV show you'd like to see. Too many people place health and fitness too far down on their list of priorities. If there happens to be time, then they'll do it. The fact is, no one *has* time. People *make* time. You just have to want it badly enough.

Be Realistic

In order for you to succeed in accomplishing your goals, it's critical for your plan of action to be one you will be able to follow through on. When people establish overly idealistic action plans, ones that are extremely difficult to adhere to, they tend to become discouraged, feeling they have failed by not staying on track. They tend to give up easily, most often as a result of frustration. To prevent this from happening to you, be honest and realistic from the start with what you are capable of doing. Err on the side of caution to avoid being overly ambitious.

It may seem you are being too cautious, but as goals are achieved in succession, you can quickly assess how wrong—or right—you've been about your goals for yourself. After all, I'd rather plan to exercise less and be pleasantly surprised that I can handle more than I thought, than plan to exercise more, much more, and be disappointed not to have as much stamina as I thought I did.

Instead of planning to be up at the crack of dawn to jog a marathon every morning, for instance, plan on starting with a brisk fifteen-minute walk to and from work three times a week. Instead of planning to do strength training two hours every night for thirty days straight, start with a routine that covers all the major muscle groups in thirty-five minutes, twice a week.

After one month, when you have assessed the situation and determined you're ready for more, bump it up a notch. For your walking routine, increase the amount of time walking from work to twenty-five minutes and/or increase the frequency to four and eventually six walks a week. For strength training, increase your number of workouts to three times a week. (See Chapter 17 for more ideas on program options for strength training.)

Envision

Always remember that wherever the mind goes, the body will follow. For each of the things you have accomplished in life (college or high school degree, a promotion, a career path, owning a car or home), chances are you envisioned what it would be like to achieve each of the those things prior to even taking action. Be sure to practice your visualization skills for health and fitness as well. This is a most powerful tool in attaining a more youthful existence because you can only manifest that which you can visualize. Hold a picture of the new you in your mind's eye, and focus on it as frequently as possible.

Avoid beginning an exercise program simply for the sake of it, or merely because your doctor said to do so. In cases like these, exercise will quickly become excruciating drudgery, and your efforts will be doomed to failure because you never envisioned any goal of yourself getting healthier in the first place. Instead, get excited about what exercise can do for you, for your quality of life, and for your life's duration. Look at physiques and figures that inspire and excite you. Then picture yourself looking your absolute best. Relive how it feels to be young again. Imagine how exciting it would be if you could feel, from within, a firm body with more power, strength, and vitality . . . more than you've had in years, decades—or ever.

To be more youthful, first believe it's possible. Envisioning—visualizing—is nothing more than believing in a successful result prior to taking action. It entails holding an image in your mind's eye. Keep in mind the self-help adage, "If it can be conceived and believed, it can be achieved." Visualizing, on a deep and meaningful level, how it felt being ten or twenty years younger is a powerful motivational tool. It is ultimately the mindset (and *heartset*), and not your chronological age, that determines how youthful you can be.

Be Persistent

Here's where short-term goals help you stay on track. Being persistent is a key element to long-term success. It is through persistence that you can accomplish much over the long term. A little bit of change performed on a regular basis will make for major advances over time. Sadly, the problem for most of us is a decided lack of persistence. Many people feel as though they've been on a diet all their lives because, well, they probably have . . . on and off and on again. The good news is that with the appropriate modifications to your nutritional plan, you will never have to diet again.

Sadly, I have witnessed too many cases where people, in a frenzy of enthusiasm or in a desperate drive to become more shapely in a brief period of time, have joined a gym, hired trainers, and worked out for two to four hours every day of every week, obsessed with how they were going to change their bodies and overhaul their lives. But then, four weeks later, they quit, never again showing up for a workout . . . until eleven months later, when desperation set in as a result of their bodies regressing from neglect and the frenzy resurfaced.

On the other hand, I've seen people come to a gym excited, but not crazed, and begin a sensible routine that had them working out with weights two to three times a week, and doing aerobic activities three to five times a week. But they were never in the gym for extensive periods of time, and they never appeared obsessed with conquering their less healthful habits. They were determined to make positive changes a permanent part of their lives, step by

DO YOU BRUSH YOUR TEETH?

Let me ask you a question—do you brush your teeth every day? (I'm certain you answered YES.) If your teeth are perfectly fine, why not give up on toothbrushing for a while? Have you ever considered that? Probably not. Why? The answer is quite simple: You know there would be consequences, both short- and long-term. After just one day, other people would begin to notice . . . every time you'd turn their way as you speak. Then, other issues would start to arise, such as cavities, gingivitis, and the need for root canal. A longer-term, more deadly, risk would be the potential for general infection, which could become quite serious, if not fatal. Everyone knows that toothbrushing on a consistent basis is absolutely essential.

For different reasons, physical activity and exercise are much the same. Without consistent effort, the body will begin to decay, bringing on many consequences, both short-term (depressed feelings, diminished strength, slower thinking, sluggishness, etc.) and long-term (increased chances for cancer and heart disease, weakened heart, weaker joints and muscles, etc.). Always remember the basic premise that *the human body was designed to be in motion.* Without persistent effort to challenge the body—to exercise and be active regularly—the body will quickly begin to break down and become vulnerable to a host of debilitating, deadly scenarios.

step. With time, they increased the intensity and frequency of their workouts, in accordance with their respective increases in strength and endurance.

One of my personal secrets to becoming leaner and stronger (for my clients, as well as myself) has been to avoid overdoing my workouts while, at the same time, never allowing obstacles to interfere with the steadiness of my routine. Whether on vacation or in the midst of the holiday season, there will always be a way for you to squeeze in at least *some* time for challenging exercise.

During more hectic periods of life, you can always abbreviate your workouts. But there is never a reason to completely eliminate them. Be sure to always incorporate at least two strength workouts every week of the year. And be mindful that there are cumulative benefits, ranging from muscle maturity (increases in muscle strength, tone, and definition) to reinforced immune systems. (Research is showing that people who exercise regularly will, over time, increase their antioxidant levels).

Not Too Little—Not Too Much

Gym acquaintances often tell me they stopped training for long periods of time. When I ask them whatever for, invariably their reason is that they simply don't have the time to do their usual workouts of one to two hours.

There are several problems with this. For starters, working out for more than seventy-five minutes at a time is *counterproductive*. There are hormonal and energy-storage considerations that cause long workouts to be less effective, not to mention the fact that there is an increased potential for injuries related to overtraining. (See Chapter 9 for more details.)

Secondly, it is possible to have a great workout in a fraction of the time you usually do it in, provided this is done on a temporary basis. A *brief* workout is significantly better than *no* workout, and the all-or-nothing approach needs to be avoided at all costs. Twelve years ago, I personally got trapped in this mindset. If I had less than an hour to complete my workout, I would skip it that day, consequently missing numerous opportunities for staying more fit. Now, I seldom miss a workout. If time is limited, then I'll just work my biceps, chest, or abdominals. When all is said and done, I feel better having done *something* than I would have doing *nothing*.

If all you have is thirty, or even twenty, minutes to exercise, don't skip it because you believe it's not effective. Every little bit of effort adds up. With my own fitness program, I sometimes have no choice but to work out between client appointments, which ends up giving me a time frame of thirty minutes or less. By the time I change into my exercise gear and do my warm-up, I'm left with about twenty minutes to actually exercise. In that time, I usually choose one muscle group and train it intensely, resting for shorter periods between sets.

Another option is to do *supersets*—say, between biceps and triceps. Supersets involve working two opposing muscles by alternately performing one set for each, back to back, prior to resting between sets. **A word of caution**: Supersets are more intense than standard routines and should not be applied to every workout.

Getting Started—*Just Do It*

The toughest part of beginning a workout routine is *just getting started*. It's that first step that seems to be the hardest, but I assure you, once you take it, you'll want to take another, and another, and another, and . . . you get the point. It's not just the physical momentum that keeps you going, either, it's also the emotional. When you start moving, you'll begin to feel an increase in energy and mental alertness, and a heightened sense of well-being overall.

Even though I love to work out—and even armed with both the scientific and anecdotal knowledge of each workout's endless benefits, physically, mentally, and emotionally—I often struggle to get my workouts started. Generally my excuses fall into one of two categories—either I had a long day of work, or I just feel lazy and want to go straight home and sit on my glutes. On those occasions, I always promise myself I'll work out for just fifteen minutes, and if I don't feel better by the end of that time, I tell myself I'll simply pack my bags and leave. Fifteen minutes is, after all, much more palatable than sixty or ninety minutes, my average workout times.

As it turns out, I almost *never* leave—not until an entire workout has been completed. In fact, there have been many times I started exercising while feeling tired, but once those endorphins started to flow, I magically began to feel more energized and ended up exercising with intensity, power, and vigor.

In fact, I almost always end up feeling much more invigorated and enthusiastic after (and even during) my workouts than if I had simply gone home after work. Over the past ten years, I can recall only two occasions when I left the gym ten minutes after starting a workout. One time, I was experiencing flu-like symptoms. The other, I was simply fatigued from sleep deprivation. (Even here there is a lesson: If your body is telling you to stop, listen to it.)

If you don't exercise because you have no energy after work, then you need to recognize one vital factor—except for the remote possibility of a medical condition, the most likely reason for feeling tired is, in fact, that you don't exercise. Seems ironic, doesn't it? Actually, it's not.

The fact is, the human body—*your* body—*needs* to be in motion. It was designed to *move*. When you move, there are a multitude of internal changes, hormonally and chemically, which lead to higher levels of energy, along with a heightened sense of well-being, enhanced psychological feelings, and a stronger immune system. So the converse is actually true: You're not feeling too tired to work out, you're feeling too tired *not* to work out. (How's that for reverse psychology?)

In summary, before you start your exercise program, you'll need to establish your goals, P-R-E-P yourself, and *just do it*. And there's one more thing—enjoy the process.

5

Optimal Nutrition for a Youthful Life

Apparently, there is a lot of confusion about knowing how best to fuel the body. What further exacerbates the problem is the endless stream of fad diets, diet centers, and diet pills which people are quite literally fed on a daily basis through ads on television and the radio, as well as in magazines and newspapers, and on the Internet. In some ways, they cause as many misconceptions as supposed benefits. To clear up this persistent state of confusion, I will go over some basic principles of nutrition. (Don't worry, you don't have to be a nutritionist to understand these basic concepts.)

On a very simple level, the food you put in your body acts the same as the fuel that's put in your car. If you use cheap gas, two things happen—performance will deteriorate and engine life will no doubt be shortened. Few people, however, apply this same logic to their bodies.

Wherever I go, I observe the kinds of food people eat. It is disappointing to see how many people (particularly the overweight) select extremely poor food options—foods that are deep-fried, slathered in butter or cream, or simply overprocessed, and offering little, if any, nutritional value. Just days before writing this chapter, I overheard two people at lunch discussing how frustrated they were at not being able to lose weight, all the while eating fried chicken wings, French fries, and pork fried rice, and drinking sugar-loaded soft drinks.

Clearly, the educational approach to good health has gone awry. Humans are the only species on earth (at least in the contemporary Western world) that eat what outside sources (TV, radio, newspaper ads) *say* to eat—the only ones on the planet who don't know what fuel is optimal in order to live longer, stronger lives of vitality (although most *do* know the best grade of gas to put in cars).

The largest, most powerful and, unfortunately, most *popular* food companies (fast-food chains and processed food manufacturers) seem to have the most influence over what Americans eat, not the nutritionists or federal agencies who have our best interests at heart. What people don't realize about all these companies is that their main mission isn't good health for you and me . . . instead, it's better financial health for themselves—the good 'ol bottom line, which usually ends up only making *our* bottoms bigger as well.

As you are bombarded by the endless barrage of glossy, enticing, cleverly packaged ads, bear in mind one very important fact of life: The human body is a beautifully designed, perfectly self-regulating mechanism, but only when it's fed what it was designed to absorb. As with a car, if the body's fuel is less than optimum, performance and longevity will diminish. And the further away from optimum you go, the more likely it is you will become weaker and more vulnerable to diseases, both internally (immune system) and musculoskeletally (muscles, joints, and overall energy flow); what follows is a decline in mental functions.

Obviously, abusing the body with alcohol, drugs, or cigarettes can lead to devastating health consequences or, to continue the car analogy, the equivalent of anything from a fender bender to a head-on health collision. But many dietary abuses, including infrequent meals and eating food loaded with simple sugars and saturated fats, are so subtle and so insidious, people aren't even aware they're cheating themselves out of a long, healthy life. Like a tire with a nail deeply embedded inside, this type of eating threatens to derail their lives somewhere down the road.

Poor diets are as destructive as substance abuse. Although poor eating habits may result in different health problems from those caused by cigarettes, drugs, and alcohol, unhealthy foods do, nevertheless, cause diseases. Whether the poison comes from the liquor store, the cigarette shop or, in smaller doses, the convenience stores and fast food drive-through lanes, America is becoming a severely malnourished nation. Even though Americans eat way too much, they often eat foods with little or no nutritional value—in sum, they are overfed but undernourished.

Before discussing the options for healthier eating, I'd like to address an urgent issue, *creeping obesity,* which often gets manipulated through top-selling books and fad diets by so-called gurus.

Beware of Creeping Obesity

To illustrate how destructive even subtle changes to your diet can be, assume that everything in your life—your activity level, your stress levels and your dietary intake—remains the same, with one exception. As a treat, you begin to drink café latte in lieu of a regular coffee . . . but only once a week. If a regular ten-ounce cup of coffee with milk, has thirty-five calories and contains one gram of fat and two grams of sugar, its latte counterpart, *Coolatta* (the leanest of the specialty coffees at Dunkin Donuts), has 210 calories for a sixteen-ounce serving that contains four grams of fat and forty grams of sugar.

This doesn't sound like much of a difference, does it? Not once a week—until, that is, you consider its long-term consequences. Over the course of a year, the extra 175 calories translates into 9,100 extra calories, or 2.5 pounds of fat. At the end of a decade, that equals twenty-five pounds of extra body fat—just for one Coolatta a week. This is what is meant by creeping obesity. What about those who drink this creamy coffee concoction two, three, four times a week? (A not uncommon habit, particularly in this fast-food, luxury-oriented society, where such coffee concoctions are as common and plentiful as the donut or coffee shops that sell them.) The results are even more noticeable, more devastating (five to ten pounds of extra fat per year) . . . again, simply from substituting Coolattas for coffees. (I haven't even addressed saturated fat or sugars, which get converted to fat more easily.)

16 oz. serving	Coffee	Coolatta (w/milk)	Vanilla Bean Coolatta
Calories	56.0	210	440
Fat (grams)	1.6	4	17
Sugar (grams)	3.2	40	69

If you were to drink just one Vanilla Bean Coolatta per week, that would add up to 21,060 extra calories a year, or six pounds of extra fat—sixty pounds at the end of one decade. Similar numbers apply for Starbucks' specialty (translated as fatty) options, including Frappuccinos. My suggestion is, if you need coffee, please avoid the fancy, trendy stuff and stick with regular coffee. It could save you from obesity and all its related diseases.

A Few Words on Fad Diets

I want you to remember three words regarding fad diets: *they don't work.* They may help you lose weight, perhaps quickly, but there are two problems with such approaches: the results are temporary, and the mostly muscle tissue, bone density, and water weight lost through such methods is the wrong *type* of weight.

With all due respect to those who are attempting, or have attempted, to get in shape through the fad diets out there today, yesterday, or even tomorrow, there is no faster, healthier way to lose weight and firm up than basic, sensible eating. This may entail the gradual, piecemeal elimination of unhealthful foods *over time.* But it should never involve the elimination or minimization of an entire food or macronutrient group, as with high-protein diets that advocate minimal to no carbohydrates.

If you have tried any fad diets, I applaud you for caring enough to want to make changes in your lifestyle. In terms of your determination, you're already on the right track. However, now is the time to redirect yourself to be on track with your actions. Positive actions combined with sincere determination *will* allow you to experience lifelong results you can never achieve through false diets and their false promises.

Once you can accept there are no magic formulas, you can move forward, developing an eating plan that is balanced, energizing, and, in many ways, healing. To prevent yourself from succumbing to even the most popular of fad diets, focus on the following three things.

1. *You need to focus on fat loss, not weight loss.* If you merely gauge yourself by general weight (which is what all weight-loss centers and fad diets do), you'll never know for sure whether you are losing fat tissue or lean tissue. After all, muscles weigh something too, and organs, brains, and bones . . . as well as water, which makes up 70 percent of your body.

2. *The human body cannot lose more than two pounds of fat per week.* If you lose more weight than that, you're also losing healthy tissue your body needs to keep, namely, bone and muscle (including the heart) tissue. It's been shown that dramatic weight losses cause even the heart muscle to weaken. Yet, one famous diet book promises that, as a result of their induction phase, you can lose thirteen pounds in two weeks. This is an undocumented claim—simply a myth.

3. *There is no such thing as spot reduction.* For example, it's impossible to

lose weight in specific areas that you choose, such as around your waist or on your thighs. The diet I just referred to also promises that the weight you'd lose would be from the mid-section. Once again, another myth. Proper eating and exercise draws on fat stores throughout the body.

The Nourishment Equation as Intended for the Human Body

Proper nutrition + exercise = well-being. That's the simple equation for optimal well-being. As you'll notice, nutrition and exercise each make up roughly 50 percent of the equation. Judging from the number of diet books on the market today and from the lack of physical activity for the average American, it appears that many people are attempting to improve their shape and their health purely from diet alone, thus satisfying only one-half the equation. But, it doesn't work that way. Nobody will increase muscle tissue and strength (or flexibility) simply by how they eat. To improve, everyone must still provide a stimulus for muscle strength. People need both proper nutrition and regular, vigorous exercise for this equation, and indeed their lives, to equal out.

As discussed in Chapter 3, diminished muscle tissue is the catalyst for many of the ailments associated with aging—excess fat-storage (with all its related diseases, such as cancer, diabetes, or heart disease), ligament sprains, osteoporosis, tendon strains, and a reduced capability for independent living, to name just a few. In order to reverse *sarcopenia* (muscle-tissue breakdown) or prevent it in the first place, muscles must be challenged (as shown in Part Two). And summoning the energy to challenge muscles requires proper fuel.

On the other side of this healthful equation, it is not enough just to exercise regularly, no matter how vigorously. If you exercise diligently, then go out and eat junk, you will never see your body's true potential for health, strength, and beauty—that's the same as giving your car a tune-up every week, then turning around and pouring kerosene into the gas tank instead of the highest-grade unleaded. Proper nourishment is equally critical. And there you have it: Exercise and nutrition are intertwined. One without the other weakens the equation to the point where optimal well-being will be virtually impossible to attain until a healthful balance is restored.

The following are basic concepts that can help you see the big picture of proper nourishment. By understanding them, you will be better able to avoid falling into the fad-diet trap.

Macro and Micronutrients

There are two categories of nutrients—micronutrients and macronutrients. My discussion here will be mainly on macronutrients—carbohydrates, fats, and proteins—the nutrients you are most familiar with.

First, however, I'd like to briefly discuss micronutrients. These are the minerals, vitamins, and elements inherent in foods, in much smaller quantities than can be found in macronutrients (examples include the minerals iron, magnesium, manganese, phosphorous, selenium, and zinc).

Most abundant when foods are in their natural form, these nutrients are necessary for the maintenance of health and the prevention of disease. The more processing a food goes through (candy, crackers, fast foods, fruit drinks, white bread, white flour, white rice, etc.), the fewer the quantity and variety of these essential nutrients. Think of it this way: You get a brand new, colorful, comfortable sweater for Christmas. It quickly becomes your favorite, but each time it gets washed, it loses some of the color and vibrancy that made it your favorite until, sometime down the line, you can hardly look at the thing. It's bleached out, has lost its form and comfort, and is ready for the rag pile. Well, that's how your stomach feels about processed foods.

Macronutrients are where most people focus their attention when considering nutrition. The three macronutrients, carbohydrates, fats, and proteins, are the primary building blocks and sources of fuel. They are *each* essential for the maintenance of basic body and brain functioning, and none of them should ever be eliminated or minimized through fad diets, or compromised by processed foods. Understanding these macronutrients, and knowing the best ways to balance and combine them, is the first step to eating wisely.

Carbohydrates

Carbohydrates serve four important functions. For starters, their main function is to provide energy for the body, particularly during exercise. In fact, carbohydrates are the most efficient source of energy for all bodily functions.

Secondly, in adequate amounts, carbohydrates help preserve tissue proteins. If the body is deprived of the right amount, there will be a reduction, or breakdown, in the body's protein levels, particularly for muscles. This would consequently lead to a reduction in lean tissue (all non-fat tissues—bones, muscles, organs, etc.) and a concomitant increase in stress to the kidneys.

A third function for carbohydrates is that they serve as a spark for fat-burning. Fat metabolism is dependent on the breakdown of carbohydrates.

Lastly, they are the primary fuel source for your brain (makes you wonder how anyone thinks optimally on a high-protein diet), and are essential for the proper functioning of the central nervous system.

Good carbohydrates/bad carbohydrates. Granted, some carbohydrates are bad for your health, but that depends on the type you choose. Carbohydrates come in two general categories, simple and complex. Simple carbohydrates tend to be processed, while complex carbohydrates are generally closer to nature. To regain or maintain youth, avoid refined, processed foods and, as with foods in general, always choose carbohydrates that are *unrefined and* unprocessed.

GOOD (COMPLEX) CARBOHYDRATES

Fruits—apples, berries, citrus, pumpkins

Vegetables—carrots, green leafy variations, and sweet potatoes

Whole grains or multi-grains (quinoa, spelt, kamut)—breads, cereals, pastas, brown rice

Another wonderful benefit derived from eating unprocessed, complex carbohydrates is that they contain *phytochemicals,* which are antioxidant compounds found in plant foods (although plants contain *some* protein, they are primarily sources for carbohydrates). Phytochemicals have been recognized by food scientists to consist of powerful disease-fighting, immune-enhancing properties.

BAD (SIMPLE) CARBOHYDRATES

Bleached cereals and processed grains, such as white rice

Fruit-flavored drinks and sweets, such as sodas, cakes, candy, ice cream, jams

White-flour bread and pasta

Simple carbohydrates have so few nutrients that if they are continually consumed over a long period of time, a number of health challenges are likely to surface, including cancer, diabetes, and hypoglycemia. Also, simple carbohydrates *do* get converted to fat much more easily than complex carbohydrates. According to the *Nutrition Almanac,* "research has shown that a diet low in pure sugar and high in complex carbohydrates has helped such problems as heart disease, high blood pressure, anemia, kidney disorders, cancer, and tooth decay."

The glycemic effect of food. In recent years, an additional measure of the quality of carbohydrates, which goes one step beyond the simple-versus-complex guidelines, is its *glycemic value* or *index* (GI). GI is defined as "an index that measures how high blood sugar rises in response to fifty grams of carbohydrates from a specific food." The standard gauge for comparison is set by a fifty-gram slice of white bread, given a GI value of 100. The lower a food is ranked in relation to 100, the healthier the food is considered to be.

The GI can be an accurate gauge if used properly. A common mistake is to judge only in absolute terms. Even authors of some well-known books on food and nutrition make this mistake (*South Beach Diet,* to name one). As with any chart or listing (including labels), to avoid being misled, it is imperative to focus on *relative value,* not *absolute value.*

As demonstrated by Terry Shintani in his book, *Good Carbohydrate Revolution,* the *glycemic load* (relative value), not the glycemic index (absolute value), is what matters most when determining the overall, relative quality of a carbohydrate. The glycemic load takes into account the caloric density of a food, and not just its weight. According to the GI, carrots (GI = 101) are higher on the scale, meaning they are less healthy than chocolate (GI = 70).

However, if you consider the fact that fifty grams of carrots have many fewer calories (21.52 calories) than fifty grams of chocolate (262.5 calories), the relative values would shift dramatically so, in reality, carrots would be much lower on the GI scale (somewhere around forty), while chocolate would rise higher (close to 100, the equivalent of white bread).

Besides not taking the caloric content of food into consideration, another problem with the glycemic index is that it doesn't measure the effect of food on insulin. When foods are measured for their impact on insulin, it becomes apparent that whole grains (brown rice, kamut, quinoa, spelt, etc.) have a much smaller impact on insulin than that measured by the GI.

Additionally, it would become apparent that high-protein foods, particularly those derived from animal sources, raise insulin to significantly higher levels than complex carbohydrate foods. According to Shintani, the GI ". . . overestimates the insulin response of whole grains and underestimates its response for refined foods, such as candy" and meats. So again, when referring to charts, be mindful of variables not reflected in mere numbers.

In order to more accurately measure how a food will affect blood sugar in real life, Shintani developed the Carbohydrate Quotient (CQ), an adjusted Glycemic Index table that incorporates the calorie density of a food; the glycemic number is adjusted downward for food with low calorie densities. It appears that "The Carbohydrate Quotient is a better predictor of insulin response than the Glycemic Index for most foods, and a better predictor of the overall healthfulness of foods in general."

TABLE 5.1. THE CARBOHYDRATE QUOTIENT TABLE

FOOD ITEM (White Bread = 100)	GI (bread)	CQ
Breads		
Kaiser roll	104	110
Melba Toast, Old London	100	122
Mixed grain bread	64	68
Stone ground whole wheat bread	61	61
White bread	100	100
Breakfast Cereals		
Cheerios, General Mills	106	118
Grape-nuts, Post	96	126
Musli, toasted	61	59
Oat Bran Cereal, Quaker	71	69
Oatmeal, old-fashioned	84	41
Oatmeal, one minute instant	94	46
Rice Krispies, Kellogg's	117	121
Special K, Kellogg's	77	80
Team Flakes, Nabisco	117	121
Buckwheat	77	46
Bulgur wheat	69	39
Cake		
Pound cake	77	118
Sponge cake	66	69
Candy		
Chocolage candy	70	97
Life Savers	100	122
Mars Chocolate Almond Bar, M&M Mars	97	129
M&M Chocolate Covered Peanuts	47	65
Cookies		
Oatmeal cookie	79	104
Social Tea Biscuits, Nabisco	79	96
Vanilla wafers	110	146
Crackers		
Graham crackers	106	129
Rice cakes	117	81
Wheat Crackers, Breton	96	132
Doughnut, cake-type	109	138
Fruit & Fruit Products		
Apple, fresh	51	42
Apricot jam	79	96
Apricots, fresh	81	66

FOOD ITEM (White Bread = 100)	GI (bread)	CQ
Cantaloupe	93	68
Dates	147	151
Grapes	61	53
Orange	61	48
Grains		
Corn	79	49
Corn chips	104	151
Popcorn	79	100
Millet	101	69
Rice, brown	79	51
Rice, specialty (mixed with wild)	79	49
Rice, white (high amylose)	80	52
Waffles, Aunt Jemima	109	94
Legumes		
Fava beans (chickpeas), boiled	47	30
Kidney beans, boild	39	27
Lentils, green & brown, boiled	41	28
Lima beans, baby, frozen	46	29
Muffins		
Muffin, plain	89	96
Oat bran muffin	86	84
Pasta		
Fettucini, egg-enriched	46	34
Spaghetti, Duram	79	59
Spaghetti, white	59	44
Spaghetti, whole-wheat	53	37
Vermicelli	50	42
Sugars		
Fructose	33	41
Glucose	139	171
Honey	104	113
Sucrose (table sugar)	93	115
Vegetables, Root		
Beets	91	31
Carrots	101	41
Parsnips	139	77
French fries	107	98
Potato, baked	121	72
Potato, new	89	49
Potato, sweet	77	49
Yams	73	49

Data from Dr. Terry Shintani's *The Good Carbohydrate Revolution*, 2002.

Fats

Over the years, fats have gotten a bad rap. While I caution against the overuse of fats (much as I caution against the overuse of just about everything), there are three main functions for fats. First, they provide the body with the largest source of potential energy. To that end, they are the most concentrated source of energy from foods—there are nine calories of energy per gram of fat (as compared with four calories each per gram of carbohydrates and protein). During rest, fats provide up to 80–90 percent of the body's energy demands. During activity, fats fuel the body for longer periods of time—up to seventy-five times longer than carbohydrates.

A second function for fats is to act as cushioning, protecting vital organs (heart, liver, kidneys, brain, etc.) from trauma. Thirdly, fats serve as an aid to thermal regulation, keeping vital organs warm. Side benefit: Fats also happen to be beneficial for maintaining healthy skin and nourishing the scalp for healthier, shinier hair.

Good fat/bad fat. Consuming dietary fats is absolutely essential for staying alive and functioning optimally. However, having too many—easy to do with the Standard American Diet (SAD)—can lead to numerous problems. To avoid that, two things are important.

1. Consume fats in moderate amounts (roughly 20 percent of total daily caloric consumption, as opposed to the typical 35–50 percent range).

2. Choose healthier fat options. Minimize unhealthful *saturated fats,* and switch to *unsaturated fats* instead. Saturated fats tend to clog arteries and that contributes to heart disease. Even worse than saturated fats are trans fats. Hidden trans fats are poisonous fats which

> **Good (Unsaturated) Fats:**
> Fish oils, flaxseed oil,
> grapeseed oil, olive oil
>
> **Bad (Saturated) Fats:**
> Butter, cheese, lard, margarine

should be avoided entirely. While I am in no way a fan of saturated fats, they at least raise the good cholesterol as well as the bad. Trans fats lower the good cholesterol and raise the bad—a double whammy.

A very simple way to distinguish between good and bad fats is by observing the fat at room temperature and seeing whether it is liquid (unsaturated) or solid (saturated).

Protein

The primary function of protein is to maintain and repair muscle and other tissues; it is essential for growth and development at any age. Protein makes *hemoglobin,* which carries oxygen throughout the human body, and it forms antibodies to fight infection and disease. Protein also produces hormones and enzymes that regulate bodily functions, and it acts as a source of energy if an insufficient amount of carbohydrates and fats have been consumed.

Proteins are made up of twenty-two distinct amino acids, most of which are manufactured by the human body. Of the twenty-two, nine cannot be manufactured. These are referred to as *essential amino acids.* It is for these nine that humans need to consume proteins through foods. For a food to be categorized as a *complete protein,* it must contain all the essential amino acids. Protein sources that contain low amounts of one or more of the essential amino acids are categorized as *incomplete proteins.* Complete proteins are found in all animals and their by-products—cheese, eggs, and milk.

Good Proteins: Hard-boiled eggs, lean beef, seafood, white meat chicken and turkey (preferably organic, wild, and free-range, respectively)

Bad Proteins: Bacon, frankfurters, hamburgers (particularly fast-food varieties), sausages

As a side note, however, I must mention—at the risk of sounding un-American —I believe that dairy (milk and cheese) was not meant for human consumption, at least not after the weaning years. Infants have a digestive enzyme that helps them break milk down properly, but this enzyme is lost past the weaning phase. And there is an abundance of research showing that milk can cause more harm than good, and can contribute to ailments ranging from cancer (breast, ovaries, prostate) to osteoporosis. I know, you're probably shocked to see osteoporosis included. Although milk is high in calcium in a glass, once inside the body, the biochemistry needed to break down this highly indigestible form of protein causes a net loss in calcium. Part of the blame is due to milk's high level of phosphorous (more on this in my *next* book). In the interim, if you're curious, visit the website, www.MilkSucks.com.

Vegetables and fruits are considered incomplete protein sources. Yet, through proper food combining, it is possible to consume complete proteins without the use of any meat sources. The key is to consume all nine essential amino acids through the food combinations you select. Particularly for vegetarians, it would be ideal to refer to a detailed breakdown of amino acids. One such list exists in the *Nutrition Almanac*. The information gathered from this chart can then be applied to the food composition table at the end of that book.

Some examples of ideal food combinations include the following: Beans and rice; peas and wheat; whole grains and sunflower seeds; beans and corn; and cereals and legumes.

Optimal Balance

Finding the optimal balance for our intake of macronutrients has lead to a major battle in dietary philosophies, separating those who believe in high-carbohydrate consumption from those who believe carbohydrates should be avoided at any cost, much like the plague. In fact, some of these fad-diet fanatics may even go so far as to blame carbohydrates for *causing* the plague.

Particularly in the past decade, carbohydrates have been accused of being the evil cause of all our health and weight problems. For many people, the obnoxious nickname c-a-r-b became the nutritional equivalent of a four-letter curse word. On numerous occasions, as I would eat a slice of multigrain bread at the gym, a fellow member would point and say, "Huh? You're eating *bread*?" while maintaining a disgusted look (as if I was biting the head of a bat), all the while thinking to themselves that I was not a true fitness professional or didn't know what I was doing.

Carbohydrates have been in the middle of a dietary battlefield, with some suggesting that as much as 70 percent of calories should come from them, and others recommending their complete elimination. Now, I know most of you probably avoid extremes, but with foods, it doesn't take extremes to throw your body's energy system off balance.

OPTIMAL MACRONUTRIENT BALANCE

Carbohydrates. 55–65 percent—the low end of the range is for overweight people, the high end of the range is for endurance athletes/participants

Fats. 20–25 percent, from superior sources, such as essential fatty acids

Proteins. 15–20 percent—the high end of the range is for strength athletes/participants

For more vitality and healthful living, it's important to have an ideal balance of *all* three macronutrients (carbohydrates, fats, and proteins). During the low-fat, high-carbohydrate heydays of the 1980s and 90s, people believed that as long as they weren't eating fat, then the food was okay, even if they were eating sugar-laden fat-free apple pie or cookies (and often dozens at a time). This led to an extreme situation where people were not watching the quality of their carbohydrate intake and were, at the same time, eliminating essential fats, an unhealthy scenario under anyone's microscope.

Then, with the subsequent rise of high-protein diets, the pendulum swung in the opposite direction. The problem with these diets is that they never distinguish between good and bad carbohydrates. The authors of such diets used *bad* carbohydrates as their only example and, therefore, condemned *all* carbohydrates for those unhealthy options, in essence, throwing the baby out with the bath water. What they failed to mention was that there are many, very healthful, essential carbohydrates and that there are some very unhealthful proteins and fats.

Once you understand what each of the three macronutrients are, and what foods provide us with those particular nutrients, the next question to answer is, "What is the optimal balance of those nutrients?" Here's where the real conflict originates in the endless debate between the high-protein/high-fat advocates and the high-carbohydrate believers.

While high-protein advocates would recommend a high-protein intake of anywhere from 40–60 percent of the diet, fats in the range of 30–40 percent, and carbohydrates as low as 20 percent (depending on whose book you're reading at the time), research has consistently shown the optimal ratio of carbohydrates, fats, and proteins to be roughly 60–20–20. In other words, 60 percent of the calories you consume should be derived from carbohydrate sources (with a range of 55–65 percent), 20 percent of your calories should come from fats, and another 20 percent should be from proteins.

It's Not Just about Calories—Carrots versus Chocolate

Two essential factors for healthful eating are the quantity and the quality of your calories. I often have this debate with Irving, a client who believes it's merely a matter of calories in and calories out. In other words, Irving believes solely in what is referred to as the *energy balance* of eating, which states that as long as you burn more calories than you eat, you will be lean and healthy.

There is one significant problem with this view, however. It does not take into account the variety of unhealthy foods available in the SAD diet, foods providing what is referred to as empty calories These are calories that do not provide much, if any, nutrient value and, thereby, get easily stored as fat. While the calorie-in/calorie-out equation might have worked for our prehistoric ancestors, it is no longer relevant for those living in what I call the Convenience Store Era—for instance, compare 1,000 calories of fast food, cakes, and processed chips with 1,000 calories of vegetables, fruits and whole grains.

More specifically, I want to use the earlier comparison between carrots and chocolate from the section on the glycemic index, where I referred to calorie density simply to demonstrate that, even in terms of the glycemic effect of food, carrots are healthier than chocolate. Now, however, I'd like to point out that calories alone are not enough of an indicator on such vital health issues.

A carrot contains many more nutrients and much more fiber than chocolate could possibly embody. In feeding the body's cells with more nutrients, your body becomes healthier and more energized. Since a chocolate bar doesn't provide many nutrients, the body will remain dissatisfied, ever hungrier for more nutrients in an endlessly vicious cycle that will result only in a continuous quest for empty calories. While the fiber in the carrot will provide a sense of satiety, the sugar in the candy will make you hungrier or crave more sweets. And so it is with all healthier foods. Feed your cells and your body will have fewer cravings, if any.

How to Eat

Not only do you need to pay attention to *what* you eat, you also need to be mindful of *how* you eat. Too many times, people inadvertently starve their bodies. They either skip meals intentionally, or they accidentally forget to eat due to a hectic work schedule or lifestyle. In either case, this is counterproductive for good health and a shapely body.

Timing Matters

Whenever anyone goes into starvation mode (not eating for over four or five hours), they end up dramatically slowing down their metabolism—their ability to burn calories. Also, to keep the body functioning, the body begins to break down muscle tissue for energy. You might think the trade-off between the short-term weight you lose is worth the long-run downside, but this will ultimately slow your metabolism down permanently, since muscle tissue is what keeps it elevated. And this slowdown will lead to an excess accumulation of fat tissue over time.

As mentioned earlier, the traditional three-square-meals approach to eating is as unhealthy as the habit of skipping meals. It was set up when this country was primarily an agrarian culture, with farmers only able to eat in the morning, at night, and once during the day when they had to stop working to fuel up. Instead, people should be eating a minimum of four, preferably five to six times a day. I'm not suggesting you eat more calories, I'm saying it is better to eat the same amount of calories over more meals. (Or, if you are overweight, eat fewer calories over more meals.)

For example, if you typically eat breakfast at 7:00 AM, lunch at 12:00 PM and dinner at 7:00 PM., you can eat less (say roughly 100–200 calories) at lunch and dinner, and add two snacks in between the main meals. In other words, have breakfast at 7:00 AM, a snack at 10:00 AM, lunch at 1:00 PM., a snack at 4:00 PM, and dinner at 7:00 PM. Of course, by snack, I don't mean candy, cookies, cake, or even frozen yogurt (too high in simple sugars). I mean real food, such as fruit, organic wholegrain cereal or toast, leftover lunch salad, or a baked yam.

I can't stress enough the need to avoid falling into the trap of skipping meals, particularly when it comes to breakfast. Your metabolism for the day is greatly influenced by how soon you eat after waking up in the morning. To burn fat, you need to eat more frequently. As a trainer for two decades, interacting with hundreds of people every week, it has become apparent that the leanest, shapeliest, most toned people are those who eat four or more times a day. On the other hand, the people who are heavier tend to skip meals or eat only twice a day.

Pre- and Post-Workout Meals

What you do before and after your workout is almost as important as what you do during it.

It never ceases to amaze me how some people at the gym eat a meal—a sandwich, a wrap, or even a yogurt—just prior to working out. And while they're still chewing, they are already beginning to walk over to the exercise area. The mere sight of this causes me to feel muscular fatigue, sometimes even nausea.

If only they understood . . .

After eating a meal, the body needs the blood to flow to the digestive organs so it can work its magic. During exercise, however, it's the muscles that require an increased blood flow in order to perform their special work. So, a dilemma results. Both the digestive organs and the exercising muscles end up competing for the same blood flow, which results in sub-optimal functioning for *both* vital systems. To avoid this and maximize the effects of each workout, here are my secrets.

Pre-workout nutrition. There are two key points for pre-workout meals.

1. Eat two to four hours prior to workout time (ideally three hours).

2. Eat a meal consisting primarily of complex carbohydrates—roughly 100 grams—with some protein (the ideal ratio of carbohydrates to protein is four to one).

As indicated earlier in my discussion of macronutrients, and as mentioned in Chapter 1, Myth 8, complex carbohydrates are the best source for energy. Some excellent examples include vegetables (such as yams and broccoli), brown rice, and wholegrain breads and cereals. Depending on how far in advance of my workout I am eating (three hours is ideal), I have several options for myself, each of which work well for providing the energy I need.

If it's three or four hours in advance, I'd either have chicken with mixed vegetables and brown rice, or a huge tossed salad with a variety of vegetables, along with sunflower seeds, walnuts, and one or two hard-boiled eggs. The dressing would be olive oil and balsamic vinegar. If it's only two hours prior, I'd have a veggie burger on whole wheat bread, with lettuce, tomatoes, bean sprouts, roasted red peppers, plus ketchup. You decide what works best for you. Just keep it healthy and wholesome.

• Without sufficient carbohydrates, exercise performance will decline. The next time you see someone drinking a protein shake just prior to their workout (I see this far too often), you'll know the consumer has fallen prey to a misconception that will interfere with the quality of their own workout, despite the bulging muscles of the model on the side of the bottle.

The primary purpose of protein is for the growth and repair of body tissues. Also, protein sources boost the metabolism more than carbohydrates and require more time to be digested and assimilated. Consuming a meal that consists primarily of protein prior to a workout would, therefore, cause muscular fatigue more readily. Conversely, complex carbohydrates provide the fuel needed by the muscles for work. Weight training is essential for the strengthening of muscle tissue and the permanent elevation of metabolism. In order to work out with greater energy and intensity, complex carbohydrates, mixed with some protein, should be consumed prior to working out.

Post-workout nutrition. Another problem with meals and workouts is what people do afterward. Some eat junk food, some eat too little, while others don't even eat at all. For the body to sufficiently recover from workouts and grow in strength, the cells and the muscles must be fed. By neglecting this crucial nourishing time, the muscles will, instead, go into breakdown. After workouts, there are two windows of opportunity to eat so the muscles can recover properly and grow in strength. Here are some tips on how to enhance the benefits of the workout just completed:

Within the first ten to twenty minutes, have simple carbohydrates (fruit-based)—preferably liquid—mixed with some protein. A natural fruit juice with protein powder is ideal. Just as with the pre-workout meal, the ideal ratio of carbohydrates to protein is four to one. Also have vitamin C (1000 mg) and E (400 IU) to enhance your recovery.

One hour later, eat a meal that consists primarily of complex carbohydrates mixed with some protein. One of my favorite choices is mixed vegetables with chicken and brown rice. Another is wholegrain pasta with seafood or a turkey burger. The meal following that, whether three hours later or the next day, should consist of a higher volume of proteins.

In order to easily take advantage of the first window of opportunity, you may want to keep healthy snacks (e.g. natural fruit juice and protein powder, bananas, raisins) in your locker for quick access after workouts. Again, for muscle recovery to begin, this window is in the initial ten to twenty minutes after completing the last exercise of your workout.

Always remember, nutrition is half the equation in the formula (nutrition + exercise) for success. If you ever need to treat yourself (cheat), be sure to avoid doing it with your pre- and post-workout meals.

The Need for Supplementation

As you've already learned, the old rules don't apply. Be it the calorie-in/calorie-out equation or the no-carbohydrate/low-carbohydrate battle, times change and so do eating habits. Today, more and more people work harder and longer than ever before. As a result, they're busier, hungrier, and more gym-happy than as recently as one generation ago. Since it's not always feasible to have a well-balanced meal, or the appetite is no longer what it used to be (as is the case with many seniors), supplementation will be helpful.

Another issue is the challenge that the toxic environment imposes on the food supply. From polluted air and toxic waters to depleted topsoil and excessive use of pesticides and herbicides, it has become nearly impossible to consume a well-balanced diet. As mentioned in Chapter 1, Myth 11, this, coupled with the destruction of the top layers of topsoil, has diminished (if not eliminated) numerous micronutrients and elements necessary for totally nourishing foods.

Supplements to Consider

In addition to consuming vitamins C and E as part of your post-workout snack, consider a multivitamin for daily consumption. For faster absorption of proteins immediately after workouts, include protein powder in your post-workout snacks. Be sure to choose only the healthier options—whey is ideal. Also, avoid powders with added sugar; look instead for protein powders with stevia.

I personally prefer using stevia for teas and coffees. While the Food and Drug Administration (FDA) does not recognize stevia as a sweetener, it has been used for sweetening beverages and foods for decades by China, Japan, and other Asian countries, and for centuries by such countries as Brazil and Paraguay. Although 250–300 times sweeter than sugar, no adverse effects have been uncovered from the consumption of stevia. It is, after all, absorbed much more slowly than many other carbohydrates, thereby stabilizing blood-sugar levels and providing for longer-lasting energy.

If your joints ache due to injuries or arthritis, glucosamine sulfate is an excellent supplement. Check with your doctor (provided she or he is up to date on the latest in nutritional research) or a nutritionist, first. A blood test would be ideal to determine whether there are any pre-existing vitamin imbalances, and, as with any other recommendation I make in this book or others you might read, do your research before you feed your body. One book I do recommend for a thorough overview of supplements is *The Best Supplements For Your Health.*

Due to a temporary rise in free radicals resulting from exercise, I believe in consuming vitamins C and E, as antioxidants, to offset any potential damage and enhance recovery from workouts. Some research shows, however, that people who exercise regularly have inherently higher levels of antioxidants. I still prefer to cover my bases.

6

Assessing Your Health and Fitness for a New Beginning

There is a helpful saying I use with all my new clients: *To get to where you want to be, first know where you're at.* It may sound overly simple at first, but think about it. How will you ever know triumph or achievement if you don't know your baseline or starting point?

By now, it's clear that you're motivated to improve your health, shape your body, perhaps even to lose some (or many) extra pounds. For a small number of you, your goal may even be to gain weight (add bulk, or increase musculature). But no matter what your physical destination, to get to where you want to be, you should know where you are currently at as a starting point—a baseline measurement to compare with, and improve from. This, in concert with the goals you've set, will help you attain your goals more easily.

Before starting, however, it would be helpful to determine your baseline measurements. It may sound unpleasant at first, but taking measurements now holds a host of benefits for the future. First of all, it will help you determine the progress you've made—or lost, in which case you'd be better able to redirect yourself. Secondly, it can serve as a motivational technique to help you stay on track. Nothing is more motivating than measuring progress as a result of your efforts. Of all the gauges you may be concerned with, the three most important ones are *blood pressure, heart rate,* and *body-fat percentage*.

With Exercise, There's More than Meets the Eye

Many people measure progress in pounds, which, as I've repeatedly mentioned, is one of the benchmarks drummed into their brains by the media. So, in addition to how much you weigh, don't lose sight of the fact that prolonged health and longevity should be the ultimate goal, particularly as you age.

Therefore, as you commence any exercise program, it is important to keep track of your blood pressure and heart rate, at rest and while exercising. The readings during exercise are important because individuals with similar readings at rest will react very differently once activities have begun, particularly intense activities.

It may help you to think of it this way: You can line up three identical looking cars at a red light and they'll all be resting at 0 miles per hour, but once the light turns green and the pedals hit the metal, all three will likely accelerate at different rates, depending on a number of variables, including the skill level of each driver (your fitness level), the fuel used in the car (what you eat), and the level of maintenance (your baseline health).

To be extra safe, it may be ideal to consult a cardiologist for a *submaximal stress test*. If you are a man over forty-five years old, or a woman over fifty, or if you've simply been sedentary for six months or more, I would highly recommend that you consider such a test. Stress tests will likely pick up any potential problems that may result from a sudden increase in sustained physical activity. They are also ways to quantify any individual's susceptibility to coronary heart disease.

While physical activity is the most natural and powerful form of preventive and rehabilitative medicine, you should still be certain there are no pre-existing maladies that could surface as a result of the exertion from exercise. You should also know if limits need to be placed on what's known as the *intensity variable*. A sudden burst of exercise and activity for any individual who has been sedentary, and who has undetected coronary heart disease, can negatively strain the cardiovascular system.

As you get more involved with your new fitness routines, your heart will become stronger and function more efficiently. This would result in lower blood pressure and heart rates, whether at rest or during activity. When this occurs, you will be able to increasingly challenge your body's duration and intensity, both of which will, in return, bring on even greater results. Hence, you and your body are rewarded with an upward spiraling positive regeneration—reversing some or many of the aging effects you may have been experiencing.

Heart Rate Measurement

Keeping track of your heart rate is relatively easy. There are two ways to measure this simple but vital reading. One is through palpation of your arteries, which can be done at one of several sites: The radial pulse (at the wrist, just to the outside of your forearm tendons), the carotid (on the side of the esophagus—wind pipe), or the temple of your forehead. Be sure to avoid using your thumb—it has a pulse of its own and will confuse any readings. Instead, use your three middle fingers.

Once you have found your pulse, count the number of beats for fifteen seconds; multiply that number by four to get your heart rate in beats per minute. The disadvantage to this method is that even if your pulse is easy to read at rest, readings are much more difficult during exercise, particularly during such activities as jogging or even walking.

A simpler alternative is to purchase a *heart-rate monitor.* My favorite is the type with a strap (which contains a transmitter) that goes around the chest, and a watch, which is a receiver. All you have to do to obtain your heart-rate reading is hold the receiver watch in front of the transmitter strap for several seconds and the reading will appear on the face of your receiver watch. Not only are heart-rate monitors convenient, but, more importantly, they are accurate. Such heart-rate readings are within 1-percent accuracy of an electrocardiogram (EKG).

To help you become aware if you are exercising with too little or too much intensity, there are many formulas for determining heart-rate ranges for all ages. Most, however, are too conservative, including the most popular one, the 220-minus-age formula. Sound familiar? This formula is used on all cardiovascular exercise-machine charts and on all heart-rate charts. It is based on the theory that for each year we are alive, our heart rates slow down one beat from the maximal heart rate we had at birth, a heart rate of 220. For most people, however, exercising in a heart-rate range derived from this formula would not be challenging enough to derive maximal health gains.

Although no formula is considered 100-percent accurate, I do believe in establishing a target range purely for the purpose of having a guideline to follow. The formula I recommend is as follows: [210 – ($\frac{1}{2}$ your age)] x 0.65 for the low end of the range and [210 – ($\frac{1}{2}$ your age)] x 0.85 for the high end of the range. The *210 – ($\frac{1}{2}$ your age)* represents your *maximal heart rate* (MHR)—this is a heart rate you should never take yourself to.

For example, if you are fifty years old, prior to applying the percentages, your baseline MHR would be 210 – ($^1/_2$ of 50) or 185. For the low end of the range, the point below which you would be exercising too lightly, multiply 185 by 65 percent (0.65) to get 120 beats per minute. To estimate the high end of the range, the point beyond which you may be exercising too intensely, multiply 185 by 85 percent; the result is 157 beats per minute. Therefore, your *target heart-rate range* would be 120–157 beats per minute. As you become fitter, or if you have been exercising for an extended period of time and are healthy, with no risk factors, then bump up the lower and upper limits to 70 and 90 percent, respectively. In this case, your target heart range would become 130–167 beats per minute.

The only disadvantage to using heart-rate monitors is the cost involved. Prices can vary from $80 to over $400, depending on features and programming options. If you are new to exercise in general, or to owning a monitor in particular, my suggestion is to stay with the lower end of the range. A very good brand I have used and recommended to many clients is the Polar model. Timex is another brand you may want to consider.

Body-Fat Percentage—Throw Out the Scale (or at Least Ignore It for a While)

What's the first thought that comes to your mind when considering your baseline measurement of shape? If you answered, "to weigh myself," congratulations. You have chosen the single most popular answer in the history of humankind. Unfortunately, however, this answer is incorrect. One of the most deceptive methods for gauging progress, or health and fitness levels, is weighing yourself. As I mentioned earlier, your total body weight is just a number. It doesn't reflect the composition of your body—the ratio of lean tissue (bones, muscles, organs, etc.) to fat. The scale does not help you understand how much of your weight is fat and how much is lean (fat-free) tissue.

Years ago, whenever I missed working out for one or more weeks (I wouldn't let that happen now), I ended up losing weight. You would think my weight would have hit the ceiling, especially for the amount of food I could pack in. The tricky part is, I was actually losing some muscle mass and adding some fat. The reason for the net loss in total weight is that muscles weigh more than fat. Muscles are much denser.

Fad diets and weight-loss centers rely on this deceptive weighing gauge partly because it is so much easier to simply lose weight than to specifically lose fat tissue. If you go on a diet that restricts all carbohydrates, for instance, you will lose a lot of water weight (carbohydrates retain water—four grams of water are attached to each gram of glycogen). This, and the subsequent breakdown of muscle tissue, will certainly lead to weight loss. . . but, *not* the kind you'd like to lose. If you recall, muscles are the driving force for your metabolism, they help your body burn fat more efficiently around the clock. If you lose muscle, you are doomed to increase your stores of fat, even if your weight may have been reduced.

Therefore, to avoid being misled, consider throwing out your scale . . . or, at least burying it in your closet for a while. Use it only occasionally to make sure you're not showing *dramatic* weight gain or loss. You can refer to it in conjunction with one of the other gauges listed below, but as a general rule, I want you to leave this section with a new outlook on weight: Too much weight is as bad as too little weight, but using a standard scale as a gauge for how much you should weigh is not always accurate for your specific body type, exercise routines, musculature, etc.

Fat—It's About Much More than Mere Aesthetics

Rather than simply relying on visual, subjective opinions as to how slim or heavy a person is, objective measures need to be used to better gauge a person's health, especially your own. But, before discussing how to measure your body more accurately, I'd like to address the almost universal concept of what is ideal.

In the arena of appearances, beauty is in the eyes of the beholder. And some people prefer the big look. In fact, Rolf is a client of mine who believes that heftier women are actually healthier. He and I have had many disagreements on the ideal body type for women. In Rolf's eyes, any slim or fit woman is anorexic (even women I know to be in the optimal 20–25 percent body-fat range). Although my client was born and raised in the United States, he somehow maintains a view held in developing societies, where being overweight is associated with good health—and even success. Although there's nothing wrong with this view from an aesthetics standpoint, there's a lot wrong with it from a health perspective.

In high school, I had an obese classmate, Luigi, whose parents—immigrants from Italy—were friends of my parents. One time, when my family was at

Luigi's home for dinner, I was fed (in a semi-forced way) not one, but *two* bowls of pasta. . . as a first course in a multi-course meal. When I refused the third serving of pasta, Luigi's mom looked at me with a distraught expression as she exclaimed, "You no lika my cookeen?" And then she proceeded to say, "You too skinny! *Mangia* (EAT)!" It was at that moment I understood Luigi's source of influence, and his predicament. Years later, when Luigi and I were in our mid-thirties, I found out he had developed type 2 diabetes. Was it genetics? Perhaps it was in his blueprint from birth. However, I believe that, had he maintained better weight control (or, more accurately, better fat composition), he would probably never have had to deal with such a condition—at least not so early in life.

Partners in a relationship do the same thing with each other. For men, are you the type who likes a little extra cushy on your wife's tushy? Women, are you the type who likes a tubby on your hubby? Those traits may be personally endearing, but they do come at a cost, particularly for the latter. Extra fat is deadly, particularly when it is stored at the midsection, around the vital organs.

Not only should everyone strive to be leaner and healthier, but this view should also be shared with dear ones who should be encouraged to also become leaner and healthier. Excess fat is a storage site for carcinogens, plus, the more fat that people carry above the healthy ranges, the more they risk hormonal imbalances, which set them up for a host of diseases, including diabetes, heart disease, and many types of cancer—breast, cervix, colon, esophagus, ovary, and prostate, to name just a few. A recent study by the American Cancer Society found, in fact, that roughly 90,000 cancer deaths every year are due to excess fat. So, forget aesthetics. Instead, think from the perspective of well-being. Have your body fat measured, and then take action—eat better and exercise.

I travel around to many colleges, speaking to students on health topics. I've got to tell you it saddens me to see how the average student population has changed in just the two short decades since I graduated from undergraduate college. I see extra fat wherever I go. It's almost as though Americans have lost any perception of an ideal body-fat ratio

With all due respect to different cultural tastes, the fact remains, all human beings are subject to the same rules of biological design. So, whether you are brothers and sisters from South or North America, Africa, Europe, or Asia, you were all designed in the same manner. And if your tastes for beauty are different, that still doesn't change the harmful effects of excess fat on the body. My point is that, rather than deciding visually whether you have too much body fat, you need to measure the estimated amount.

Better Gauges of Fatness—The True Measures of Success

Despite the complexity and enormity of what I consider to be this country's battle with obesity, when the dust clears, it really all boils down to only three main methods I recommend for all my clients and seminar audiences: *body-fat composition, girth measurements, and clothes-fitting.*

Body-fat composition is the most accurate way to determine a healthful shape and it is one way to circumvent subjective views imposed by others, such as models, friends, the popular media, or even ourselves. There are numerous methods for estimating fat percentage, but I caution you ahead of time that none are 100-percent accurate. The method I prefer, based on simplicity and level of accuracy, is *skinfold* measurements (I recommend the Lange brand). This method involves the use of a device known as a caliper, which includes two prongs to measure the fat situated immediately under the skin, but above the muscle. (See "The BMI Weakness" on page 72.)

Please don't panic if this all sounds like science fiction to you at first. A trainer at your local gym or a physical therapist should easily be able to assist you. This gauge uses a pinching technique to measure fat at a predetermined number of sites on the body. I prefer using the five- and six-site formulas, for women and men respectively, since they take variations in fat distribution into account. After measuring the suggested sites, the measures are summed up and the total values are plugged into a formula or chart provided by the manufacturer.

The estimated fat percentage at each respective total skinfold sum (the total tally) rises with age. For young adults, approximately half the total body fat is deposited under the skin, while the remaining fat is internal, wrapped around organs. With age, a greater proportion of body fat is situated internally.

The most healthful ranges of body fat are the following.

Age	Up to 35	35–55	55 and up
Females	17–22%	18–23%	19–25%
Males	9–14%	10–16%	12–18%

The lower ends of the ranges are more healthful than the higher ends. Even body-fat percentages below these ranges are healthy, but within limits. There is what is referred to as *essential body fat*. A certain amount of body fat is needed for healthful living and normal bodily functioning. For women, the essential body fat is 8–10 percent, while for men it is 3–4 percent. In other words, to stay alive, women and men should not go below these respective amounts of body fat.

If, on the other hand, you find yourself above the range—by a little or even a lot—there's no need to panic. Your number (body-fat percent) is subject to change upon will—*your* will. Your goal, at least initially, should be to simply bring yourself a few percentage points closer to that range, whether you're starting out at 28- or 50-percent body fat. For each percentage point of fat you lose, the healthier you will become. The closer you get (to the range), the better you'll feel, live . . . and look. You've already taken the first step to dwindling down the number just by picking up this book—and reading it, of course.

Girth measurements are another approach to gauging your shape objectively. This is a convenient and inexpensive method of determining progress based on the notion that fat is commonly distributed at various sites on the body, such as arms, hips, thighs, and waistline. Any cloth tapemeasure will do, although, for more accuracy, I prefer the Gulick brand, which has a spring-loaded, sliding cylinder attachment that helps you to know when to stop pulling on the tape. This helps prevent taking measurements that are inconsistent and

THE BMI WEAKNESS

Although I am a firm believer in the value of body fat measurements, I am not a fan of Body Mass Index (BMI), the most popular method of estimating fat percentage. While it is easy to apply, the main reason for its popularity, it is highly inaccurate in that it relies solely on height and weight, which is vague and unreliable at best—some studies have even proven BMI to be inaccurate, and no indication of fat or lean mass can be determined through this method. Consider me as an example. After plugging my height and weight into the formula, it was determined that I am overweight. Sounds bad, right? But, when you consider the fact that my body-fat percentage is in the 6–8 percent range, you realize how irrelevant the BMI turns out to be.

smaller than the truth, particularly at sites that are softer, due to extra fat tissue.

There are two ways to apply girth measurements. One use for them is to simply keep a record of all the sites over time. This will help you determine where there may be problem areas. Another way, which requires only waist and hip measurements, is to compute your *waist to hip ratio*. Here, you simply divide the circumference of your waist by the circumference of your hips. Measure your waist at the smaller circumference of your natural waist, usually just above the navel, and measure the hips at the widest circumference of your buttocks. For women, the ratio should be below 0.86, and for men, it should be below 0.95. If your ratio is above these markers, there is an increased risk for health challenges because it's not just the amount of fat you need to be concerned about, but also the distribution of fat (see table below).

Here is a good place to point out the inconsistencies you've been bombarded with by the media, the bestselling diet books, fashion models, or diet gurus. Whether it's your BMI or fat distribution, everyone is unique. There is no one single best form of gauging fat. Some are comfortable using calipers, others would prefer tapemeasures. Bottom line—everyone is different. Your body shape, weight, musculature, height, fat distribution, and percentages are different from mine and probably from 80–90 percent of your fellow readers. So it's important to take measures accurately and objectively—only then will they be *true* measurements.

Male	Female	Waist/Hip Ratio Health Risk
0.95 or below	0.80 or below	Low risk
0.96 to 1.0	0.81 to 0.85	Moderate risk
Above 1.0	Above 0.85	High risk

A third gauge is ***clothes-fitting***. Take note of how you fit into the clothes you wore five, ten, even twenty years ago. There is no reason why you shouldn't be able to fit into the clothes you wore at an earlier age . . . unless, of course, you're in better shape now than you were then.

One word of caution, however, is to avoid the mistake of merely looking at the size number on the label. Relying on the sizes of the clothing you currently wear in comparison to what you had worn in the past will be deceptive. Clothing manufacturers have adjusted the American clothing-size charts downward several times over the past fifty years. I personally recall reading about three downward adjustments since 1980 alone.

For women, what was a size twelve in the 1950s is probably a size four now. Perhaps the purpose for such downward adjustments was to prevent consumers from feeling discouraged about their size. However, this is a serious problem, misleading people into believing they're on track even if they're not. So, if you currently wear a size six, and you wore a size six in 1980, rather than be complacent, perhaps it's time to start hitting those weights, as well as becoming more active and stricter with your nutritional intake.

About two months ago, while shopping at my favorite sporting goods store, I was shocked to find out the shirts that fit me best were actually Small. I had been wearing Large, and sometimes Extra Large, from the same manufacturer as recently as one year earlier. The Small was a blow to my ego since I've been trying to gain weight—muscle weight, that is. Yet, in my heart, I knew I was the strongest and most muscular I had been in all my life. Not to mention I was also my heaviest (again, in terms of muscle weight). So hold on to your older garments and use them as a barometer. After all, size does *not* matter—not with labels anyway.

Additional Gauges of Health and Fitness

For anyone who has already been exercising, there are other areas of health and fitness you may want to keep track of: *flexibility, muscular strength,* and *muscular endurance.*

For **flexibility**, the range of motion around a joint, there is the *sit-and-reach test*. This test primarily measures the flexibility of your lower back and hamstring muscles. The secondary muscles, the support muscles that indirectly affect your capability in this test, are your shoulder and calf muscles.

Many gyms have a sit-and-reach box. If one is not available, then simply use a tapemeasure or yardstick. Place a piece of masking tape at the twelve-inch line, perpendicular to the tapemeasure. Remove your shoes and socks and, with the one-inch line closest to you, align the heels of your bare feet at the twelve-inch point. Lightly place one hand above the other (do not clasp hands) as you take in a deep breath. Then, as you exhale, slowly lean forward as far as you can, keeping your back flat and your legs straight. Perform this test three times, resting several seconds between each stretch. Record the highest of the three scores.

For ***muscular strength***, the force that a muscle or muscle group can exert against a resistance, a common test is the one-repetition (rep) max (1-RM) test. This measures the heaviest weight that can be lifted for one rep. The one problem with 1-RM, however, is that it places an enormous amount of stress on the joints involved, particularly for people who have been inactive. A safer, modified version of the 1-RM for a given exercise, say the chest press, is to exercise with a very light weight—roughly 50 percent of your subjective predicted maximum—performing fifteen reps. Based on the amount of fatigue, or lack of it, resulting from that initial set, change the weight so that during the next set of twelve reps you experience muscular fatigue by the last three or four reps. Be sure to rest one minute between sets.

A more scientific textbook method is one which estimates the 1-RM based on a seven-ten-RM. For an untrained individual, it is estimated that a maximal weight lifted in a seven- to ten-rep set represents approximately 68 percent of his or her 1-RM ability. The estimates are higher for trained individuals—79 percent of 1-RM.

My suggestions for such a strength test is to first do a brisk, but light, *general* (aerobic) *warm-up* for six to ten minutes. Then do a *specific warm-up*. This entails using a very light weight for fifteen reps of the exercise you're about to test yourself on. Rest for one minute, then raise the weight to a point where you can perform seven to ten reps, experiencing local muscular fatigue by the last two or three reps. The following are formulas you can use to estimate your 1-RM strength levels.

If you are untrained: 1-RM, kg = 1.554 (7–10-RM weight, kg) – 5.181

If you are trained: 1-RM, kg = 1.172 (7–10-RM weight, kg) + 7.704

To convert a figure from pounds to kilograms, divide the weight by 2.2. After calculating your 1-RM, multiply that figure by 2.2 to generate the final estimate in pounds.

To measure ***muscular endurance***, which is a muscle's ability to resist fatigue or persist in physical activity, there are two common tests. One is a pushup test for the upper body and the other involves crunches for abdominals. In both cases, the key is to perform, without rest, as many reps as possible in one minute.

Doesn't sound too bad, right? But there's a catch. To measure accurately, it is important to maintain proper form with each rep. When doing pushups, keep your hands shoulder-width apart. For women, if need be, you may rest your knees on the floor. For men, only the hands and toes should touch the floor. Keep your head in alignment with your torso, avoid dropping your chin. For both women and men, maintain a straight torso, no bending at the hips or sagging at the lower back.

Once you have your baseline measures for each of the above tests, compare results every three to four months to be certain you are on track. If you made progress, congratulate yourself and consider revising some of the parameters so you can continue to progress (see Chapter 17). If you should regress at any point, simply analyze what you have done over the past few months and determine what areas need improvement, whether it's the frequency or intensity of exercise, the level of physical activity, or nutrition.

Now that baseline measures as well as goal-setting (see Chapter 4) have been covered, your course of action should be easier to establish. It's getting close to the point in your action plan where the rubber hits the road. However, before discussing actual exercises and program options, I have just a few more points to share with you, starting with a brief discussion on the power of aerobics.

The Need for Cardiovascular Conditioning

Although the main thrust of this book is to encourage you to use strength training as a tool to a more youthful lifestyle, this should not be at the exclusion of *cardiovascular* (heart and lung) *conditioning*.

As vital and comprehensive as strength training is for overall health, cardiovascular exercising also offers invaluable, life-saving, age-reversing benefits that are specific to this form of exercise. After all, the single most important muscle in the human body is the heart. And, as beneficial as strength training is for the heart, the most profound exercise for heart health is cardiovascular conditioning—aka aerobic exercise—so be sure to include both exercise modalities in your health routine.

Perhaps you can do so by picturing your health as a seesaw, always tottering in one direction or the other. As you grow more familiar with the practices and routines in this book, you'll begin having your strength days and your cardio days. This may sound like Greek to you now, but soon you'll be speaking my language, and you'll come to see that the best way to balance the seesaw of your health—and your life—is to divide your strength training and your cardio equally.

How Important Are Aerobics?

On a scale of one to ten, aerobic exercise rates about a forty-seven. There are not that many absolutes in life, but as it does with strength training, medical science backs me up with consistent reports that few things are as good for you, and in as many different ways, as aerobic exercise.

Aerobic exercising conditions the cardiovascular system (arteries, veins, heart, and lungs) by increasing the amount of oxygen available to the body. Also, such exercise conditioning enables the circulatory system to use oxygen more efficiently. It enhances aerobic endurance, muscular endurance, and exercise capacity. Performed on a regular basis, cardiovascular activities help prevent the development of heart disease and help diminish those effects if they already exist. One study showed that moderate-intensity step-aerobics conditioning significantly strengthened the hearts of people with severe chronic heart failure.

Studies have demonstrated that blood pressure, cholesterol, and triglycerides can all be reduced through regular cardiovascular conditioning, and that reductions in blood pressure occurred even in individuals already diagnosed with hypertension. One study showed that the lining of the arteries, the endothelium, remains more flexible—better able to dilate (grow and expand) to allow for better passage of blood platelets—when people are aerobically active. Loss of this endothelial flexibility, commonly associated with sedentary living, leads to *atherosclerosis* and other forms of cardiovascular disease.

Aerobics has also been shown to diminish, if not eliminate, the potential for cancer, diabetes, osteoporosis, and other major diseases. The aerobic activities most beneficial for osteoporosis are weight-bearing and higher impact activities. For this reason, swimming is not as protective of bone health, or as helpful at preventing osteoporosis as jogging, stair climbing, walking, and similar weight-bearing activities are.

What Are Aerobics?

Clearly, you can see the many advantages and benefits of aerobic exercise. But in addition to learning about burning (calories, that is), it would be helpful to delve into some more specifics about the various exercises, movements, and practices that fall under the broader umbrella term we hear so often—*aerobics*.

Aerobic exercises and activities are those which require the movement of large muscle groups (legs, arms, or both) in a rhythmical, steady pattern for extended periods of time. Aerobic activities are those which require the utilization of oxygen to generate energy from food. In order to activate the aerobic processes in the body, an exercise needs to be performed continuously for at least ninety seconds. Much like the space shuttle uses booster rockets to boost it out of the earth's atmosphere, this ninety-second kick start would get you past the carbohydrate fuel-burning phase and begin the shift toward the fat-burning phase. Carbohydrates are the fuel source for quick, powerful bursts of energy. Fats kick in as the fuel source when carbohydrates are used up (after about fifteen to twenty minutes of steady movement). For optimal cardiovascular benefits, and to reach this fat-burning phase of exercise (the *aerobic threshold*), it is necessary to move your body continuously, without stopping, for a minimum of fifteen to twenty minutes at a relatively brisk pace.

There are no absolutes at this point. This is *your* exercise program, personally designed for *your* unique body by the one who knows it best—*you*. The terms *minimum, relatively,* and *brisk* are subjective and best left up to you, but I offer them as definitions of what, exactly, constitutes aerobic movement. Please don't let them dissuade you if you're just getting started, or hold you back if you've been doing this for years. I simply offer them as a starting point so everyone's on the same page.

For optimal results, it is recommended that you exercise at an intensity that will bring your heart rate to a range of 65–85 percent of your maximal heart rate. As discussed in Chapter 6, maximal heart rate is best determined by dividing your age in half and then subtracting that number from 210—the formula is 210 minus $\frac{1}{2}$ your age.

If you're out of condition or have been sedentary for an extended period of time, it would be best to stay in the 65–75 percent range. Also, it may be better to start out exercising for bouts of ten minutes, two or three times a day, rather than pushing the envelope and doing twenty or thirty minutes at a clip. As you become fitter, raise the intensity to the 75–85 percent range and increase the length of your exercise bouts until you are able to exercise for thirty minutes or more, *without rest*. Also, increase your frequency to at least five days—and eventually seven days—per week.

That may seem like a lot right now, but the nice thing about aerobic exercise is that it can easily become a fun activity you will actually look forward to. (I know that if I have to miss a few days, or even one day, of aerobic exercise, I *really* feel it, and not in a good way.) As you increase in fitness levels and duration of exercise, your satisfaction with, and affection for, aerobic exercise will grow. You will become fonder of it and it won't feel like *seven days of exercise,* but more like *health and fitness every day.* Taken literally, those phrases may mean the same thing, but I can tell you from experience that they're quite different to your body, mind, and soul.

The key here is to challenge your body and bring it to a level just beyond what it is normally accustomed to. Challenging your body is always a major element in generating positive results from your aerobic workouts.

Think of your fitness goals as a series of finish lines you want to cross. Each time you burst through that ticker tape, be sure to move the finish line you just crossed back a little, and then farther back next time, and again the following time. You should always be pushing that finish line back, farther and farther, as your goals are reached and your body develops strength and endurance.

For instance, if you're used to walking five consecutive blocks, then walk six blocks. If you typically jog two miles in twenty minutes, try completing 2.2 miles in that time. Perform aerobic exercises and activities for twenty to sixty minutes, five to seven times per week. Vary your exercises every three to six weeks so your body and mind never get bored with the same routine. For example, if you've been taking brisk walks for the past month, then add (or switch to) bicycling. Progress plateaus when the body *adapts* to the same routine . . . and the same intensity.

Another way to gauge intensity is by applying the *talk test*. As you begin your fitness regimen, you should be able to talk comfortably while exercising. When you become more advanced, challenge yourself to the point where you are unable to easily carry on a conversation while exercising. Always start with a warm-up and finish with a cool-down (these involve doing the same activity, but at a much lighter intensity).

Examples of Aerobic Exercises

Now it's time for the rubber to hit the road again, as we start to talk about what really matters—the exercises themselves. Aerobic exercises include aerobic exercise classes, bicycling, cross-country skiing, dancing, hiking, jogging, roller skating/blading, rowing, swimming, walking, and a host of cardio machines (i.e., ellipticals, exercise bikes—upright and recumbent—stairclimbers, and treadmills). Lots of variety there, right? This should be good news. If you get bored with one type of exercise, say swimming, you can always switch to another, for example dancing.

Try not to make the common mistake of confusing sports with aerobic exercise, simply because a sport involves fast movement. When people play sports, such as basketball, handball, soccer, squash, or tennis, they believe they're getting an aerobic workout. *They're not.* These sports *do* involve a combination of aerobic (requiring oxygen due to longer duration) and anaerobic (not requiring oxygen due to short duration) energy systems. And they *do* recruit numerous muscles and require brisk movement, but because of the stop-and-go nature of these sports, they are not continuous enough to qualify as aerobics. Once you stop to serve a tennis ball or take a foul shot in basketball, your energy systems shift from an aerobic setting to an anaerobic one. Again, at least ninety consecutive seconds of movement must be continuously performed for aerobic systems to begin kicking in. And, as previously mentioned, depending on intensity, it takes fifteen to twenty minutes to reach the aerobic state.

Don't get me wrong. Sports are a fantastic way to keep your body younger, leaner, and even stronger. The stop-and-go effects of sports result in a different set of benefits from aerobics (and strength training). They force you to react quickly, keeping your reflexes sharp, while encouraging you to use multiple muscle groups synergistically, in ways the more-regimented exercises and activities cannot do. The thing to understand here is that *playing sports does not rule out the need for cardiovascular conditioning.*

It's a matter of public perception—fitness websites often picture healthy, happy, attractive people playing sports. Therefore, you might naturally think sports qualify as aerobic exercise. However, since you are well past the stage where such misconceptions can affect you, you now know that sports are good for you as well.

But back to the subject here—specific, technical, and official aerobic exercise. While such exercises (cycling, running, or swimming) are great ways to get in your aerobic workout, there are also other ways to incorporate aerobics into your daily lifestyle. For example, make walking part of your daily commute to and from work. If you use public transportation, get on the bus or train one stop past where you usually board, and get off one stop early so you end up walking an extra eight blocks or so. If you drive, park at a distance requiring you to walk at least ten minutes in each direction. Whenever possible, use stairs instead of elevators and escalators. At lunchtime, go for long, brisk walks. Or walk to eat lunch at a place that is ten or fifteen minutes away from your office—for example, a pleasant park where you can enjoy a healthy lunch you brought from home or bought at a local health food store.

It may take longer to fit in your aerobic exercise this way, but if it's the only way you can work out that day, then so be it. You may have to take into account how long it will take to walk to work from your new, more distant stop, or how much earlier you'll have to leave your own house to walk to the next stop, but just by taking a few extra minutes to plan it out, the extra steps will soon become routine—you won't be late and the benefits, in terms of your well-being and youthfulness, will add up.

In summary, if you are ever uncertain as to which activities are cardiovascular in nature, remember these three criteria needed for an activity to be classified as cardiovascular/aerobic:

1. It should engage large muscle groups

2. It must be continuous in movement (no stop and go)

3. It needs to be performed steadily for extended periods of time (fifteen to twenty minutes minimum)

Three Keys to Successful Aerobics

As with strength training, when doing aerobic exercises, there are three elements necessary for success in achieving your goals:

1. Proper technique

2. Intensity

3. Frequency

Before starting a dedicated aerobics routine for the first time, or even if you've already begun, it is vital to learn the correct techniques for exercise—for two reasons. First, by having an awareness of correct form, you will generate greater results with the same effort and, second, you will minimize your chances for injury.

Here are three basic tips that pertain to a number of activities.

1. Use the heel-ball-toe rule for jogging, running, and walking activities. Always land on your heel first, then roll onto the ball of your foot, and finally push off from your toes. This technique will help distribute the *ground reaction forces* (the reaction force supplied by the ground, through the body, in relation to the amount of force exerted by the body onto the ground) more evenly and help prevent injuries, such as shin splints.

2. For jumping activities (i.e., rope-jumping and aerobic classes), always land first on the toes and ball area, followed by the heel. This is the inverse of such forward-moving activities as jogging, running, and walking. Before jumping upward, have the entire foot touch the floor momentarily.

3. When cycling, protect both your back and your knees by positioning the seat at the proper height for your leg length. For your leg on the downstroke, there should only be a slight bend at the knee while the foot of that leg stays flat on the pedal. Also avoid positioning your seat too high as this will put extra pressure you don't want on your lower back.

With good form, you will generate faster results in a safer manner. In order for exercise to be effective, do it with the right amount of intensity. If you are interested in high-impact activities, such as jogging or running, first check in with a sports doctor, physical therapist, or kinesiologist (a specialist who understands muscle imbalances) to be sure your joints can handle the ground reaction forces resulting from each foot strike on the ground. Unfortunately, many older adults lose some degree of shock-absorbing capabilities in their joints (at the ankles, knees, and hips), and this limits their ability to perform high-impact activities safely and effectively. If this includes you, no need to fret. You can still get fantastic results from lower-impact activities, such as bicycling and power walking.

Mixing Aerobics with Strength Training

In the same way you wouldn't mix lunch and dinner, aerobics and strength training should not be done during the same workouts. When done at the appropriate intensity level, each of these requires a good amount of energy. If both are pursued with vigor in the same workout, then whichever is performed last (strength after aerobics or vice versa) will generate suboptimal results. So, for best results, keep your strength training and aerobic workouts separate. If you have no choice but to perform both in the same workout, then prioritize between aerobics (cardio) and strength training.

Where to fit in cardio exercise depends on your age and personal goals. If you are under age sixty, then cardio is a major priority. If you are sixty or older, balance and strength training become more of a priority. When to do cardio, relative to strength training, also depends on your goals. If your primary concern is to enhance your aerobic capacity, then cardio should be done at the beginning of your workouts. For all other goals (fat loss, muscle tone, strength increase, etc.), strength training should be completed first, while your muscles are at their strongest level.

If, as I warned earlier, you start to get addicted to the positive feeling brought on by regular aerobic training, you can still get your fix by walking to and from the gym instead of driving or cycling. If you work out on home equipment, build in some type of walk before or after your strength conditioning, maybe to the store for a bottle of water before you start lifting, and back again afterward to get some more.

With aerobics (and strength training), it is important to prevent *adaptation,* the point at which the body gets so accustomed to an exercise or activity that progress plateaus. In order to maintain enthusiasm for aerobic exercises and generate the best possible results from your efforts, rotate exercises and maintain intensity.

More Benefits of Aerobics

Of all forms of exercise, aerobics burn the most calories per minute. Other benefits include cholesterol and fat reduction. With running, for example, it is possible, to burn over 1,100 calories per *hour.* While that may seem like an extreme end of the spectrum, it is important to choose modalities you are most likely to stay with for the long term.

Another nice thing about aerobic exercise is that it doesn't necessarily require money or space. One of the safest, cheapest, and most convenient

DETERMINATION = SUCCESS

Jim, the father of one of my clients, had high cholesterol and high blood pressure and was diagnosed as a potential candidate for heart disease. He knew he needed to exercise to improve his health. So, with his new-found motivation, he considered his options and began walking in his home, overcoming the drawback that it was a really small Manhattan apartment. At first, he walked back and forth across his living room for ten minutes at a time, then he eventually worked up to walking for an hour. After five months of this, Jim had lost seven pounds of fat, and in the process, his blood pressure, cholesterol, and triglycerides had *all* been lowered.

Such positive changes are not unusual. What *is* unusual is that he accomplished them by walking back and forth in the living room of his small New York City apartment.

forms of aerobic exercise is simply getting out of the house and walking. And this can be done anywhere, anytime—from the moment you step out your door. Just be sure to keep your body moving continuously, for twenty minutes or more.

It can, as I said earlier, become a part of your commute to and from work, and it can be done in the park or even in your own living room. No need to step out any door—if you're motivated enough, you can achieve aerobic fitness just by walking within your home . . . whether you live in a house or an apartment. People often make excuses for not exercising, but this clearly illustrates there really is *no* excuse for not being able to exercise aerobically.

Sal's Summary

Three elements are essential in order to generate positive results: *Duration, frequency,* and *intensity.* Regarding duration, it takes roughly twenty minutes of continuous, brisk activity to reach the fat-burning stage. If this is too difficult for you, start with ten-minute bouts, two to three times a day.

Regarding frequency, four to seven days a week is ideal. And, of course, when it comes to intensity, remember to bring your heart rate to a range of 65–85 percent of your maximal heart rate.

Concentrate on the Starting Line, Not the Finish Line

Lastly, I'll remind you that while life may seem to be about crossing the finish line at times, never forget the feeling you have as you approach the starting line. New goals must continually be evolving, so that, as you reach one finish line (or goal), and then another and another, you must always be looking forward to that adventurous new sense of excitement you can feel as you walk toward another starting line, and another and another. When life is not always so centered on finishing, it's possible to truly sit back and enjoy what's really important—the *journey.*

8

Strength Training— The Light at the End of the Tunnel

Strength training is extremely beneficial to people of both genders and all ages. The really great thing about strength training is its adaptability. No matter what age, weight, or sex you are, there are specific benefits to be obtained from building strength. It is especially critical for women who have reached, or passed, their menopausal years to include this vital mode of exercise in their weekly activity schedule.

National health organizations always recommend that strength training be included in a comprehensive fitness program, and the benefits to be derived from the strength-training program taught in this book are numerous. Strength training will: decrease blood pressure and heart rate; improve blood-fat levels and functional capacity; increase connective (ligament and tendon) tissue, insulin sensitivity, metabolism, and muscle; reduce body fat; relieve low back pain; and thicken bone density. (And you thought you were just going to trim down and tone up.) Many improvements in physical function are associated with the increases in endurance, muscle strength, power, and hypertrophy that result from strength training.

Everyone knows that change takes time. But in this case, time really *is* on your side. With the right technique, the right amount of intensity, and a healthful diet, you will begin to feel significant positive changes in a short period of time. Take heart.

Changes To Be Expected in Four to Six Weeks

With the right amount of consistency, intensity, and variety, the following changes will occur, or will have begun to occur in just four to six short weeks. Some changes, as you will see, are *immediate*.

If any of the quantified changes below sounds too small or insignificant for your expectations, first consider how long you have not challenged your body in such a way. Secondly, just imagine how much more you will improve when you continue with this program beyond just four or six weeks—for twelve weeks . . . twelve months . . . twelve years.

Benefits are cumulative. They build on each other, much like compound interest on money invested. In some cases, change will be exponential. In other cases, it will simply continue to accumulate steadily with the passage of time.

- *Muscle mass will increase 6–8 percent.* As much as two decades of strength loss can be reversed after performing strength-training exercises for just two months.

- *Muscular strength improvements will exceed 22 percent in as little as four weeks.* In your first three months, you can attain strength increases of up to 38 percent, and increases of 77 percent can be achieved by the end of one year of training. One study actually showed a strength increase of 174 percent after just eight weeks of strength training for nonagenarians, people aged ninety and above. See what you've got to look forward to?

- *Stronger muscles mean stronger, thicker bones.* Strength training is the most direct and effective approach for preventing osteoporosis. In four to six weeks of following my program, you will experience a significant increase in bone density of about 0.5 percent; at the end of one year, density will increase by 1.7 percent.

- *Can you say metabolism boost?* Also related to increased muscle mass is an increase in metabolism—your body's calorie-burning engine. Muscle tissue requires more energy to be well-maintained. Fat-burning will increase by 16–23 percent.

- *Goodbye fat.* As a result of fat-burning, body fat will diminish by 2–4 percent. After six months, body fat can drop 10–15 percentage points, depending on your fat levels at the beginning of this program.

- *Through strength training, the heart becomes stronger and more efficient.* Heart rate during rest or physical activity should drop by three to five beats per minute.

- **Blood pressure will be reduced.** Although this factor continues to be debated, there are studies showing that six months of resistance training reduces systolic pressure by 8 mm Hg (hemoglobin) and diastolic pressure by 9 mm Hg. This translates into a reduction of about two mm Hg after just six weeks.

- **Cholesterol reduction.** You will experience significant decreases in total cholesterol and LDL (bad) cholesterol of 4–5 percent, and significant increases in HDL (good) cholesterol of 8–10 percent.

- **Insulin sensitivity will improve by 48 percent.** It's been found that strength training for thirty minutes three times a week increases insulin sensitivity. A single session of resistance exercise improves whole-body insulin sensitivity for up to twenty-four hours. This is a critical variable for preventing or controlling diabetes and is particularly beneficial for anyone with diabetes. Your body will be better able to control your blood-sugar levels with less insulin, thereby placing less stress on your pancreas.

- **Strength training will quickly enhance the functional capacity and quality of life for people with rheumatoid arthritis.** After six weeks of training, there will be a reduced number of painful joints, a faster sit-to-stand time, increased grip strength, and reduced nighttime pain.

- **Total weight should drop by eight to twelve pounds.** Bear in mind that, unlike unhealthful fad diets, which promise huge amounts of weight loss (up to ten pounds in one week), the weight lost through my approach is purely from diminished fat tissue, and is not due to water and lean-tissue losses.

I hope you can now see the unique opportunity afforded by my system. Not only does it work, but in relation to other programs, it works fast. Here's your chance to not only lose weight, but to do so intelligently and healthfully . . . and gain strength in the process. This all leads to a higher quality and quantity of life.

Immediate Changes

Despite the relatively rapid benefits of my program, no system is a magic bullet that makes changes overnight. Although changes in shape and strength won't be apparent for several weeks, some changes *do* occur as soon as you start.

- *Right from the instant you lift your first weight, shifts on a chemical level begin to occur.* This change occurs on a cellular level for several weeks, before the changes start becoming visible.

- *You will also experience an elevated mood, improved psychological well-being, and mental clarity.* Exercise is recognized as the most immediate and profound stress reducer known to humans. This occurs not only because exercise dissipates nervous energy, but also because it directly influences the body's relaxation response. Since the body is designed to be in motion, the moment you begin to move, a whole series of chemical and hormonal alterations begin to occur, diminishing or eliminating the tendency for depression or clouded thinking. Strength training reduces anxiety while it improves energy, morale, self-esteem, and ease in falling asleep. Studies have shown that cognitive function, such as memory, problem-solving, and reaction time, improves as well. Strength training also appears to give women a sense of empowerment. Research indicates that people who do regular exercise generally have a more positive outlook on life and they tend to confront the daily hassles of their workday world more positively than people who are sedentary. Not only does exercise *directly* create psychological benefits as a result of positive mental changes, but as a result of the positive physical changes, it also *indirectly* creates such benefits.

Overall, simply by beginning my program, you will become a happier and stronger person ... mentally, emotionally, and physically. There's no telling who you'll become if you stick with it.

The Promise

Before moving forward, it's a good idea to make a promise. Your promise to me (and yourself) actually has three parts connected to exercise, plus another that's related. First, promise you'll be persistent and stick with this program for at least four weeks. That's right, give it your best shot for twenty-eight days. Secondly, stick with the techniques detailed in Part Two. They were designed specifically for you and will only work if you follow them closely. Third, as your body adapts to your initial workout intensity and you get stronger, continually challenge yourself by increasing your workload. Finally, you should also begin following the nutritional guidelines in Chapter 5. This won't be as challenging as it sounds because, the better you feel, the better you'll want to eat.

In return, my promise to you is that, through persistence, you will see and feel noticeable changes—changes you couldn't have imagined possible. They will be real and you can measure them. You will become stronger. You will have more vitality. You will even notice some of your muscles becoming more toned. (You may also notice your clothes becoming more comfortable.) You will look and feel younger, have more aerobic and muscular endurance (for physical activities and life overall), be more mentally alert, and emotionally uplifted.

But, don't stop there. Upon reaching this stage, you will be ready for the next step, which includes adding variety and intensity to your routine. By following the guidelines in this book, you will feel, and live your life, as though you were younger. And by younger, I mean you will function as though you were ten, fifteen, even twenty, years younger.

That is why I urge you to promise me, and yourself, you'll give it those twenty-eight days—four weeks (or for those with very short attention spans, one month). The ripple effect this course of action will have on your life will be incredible, and I speak from experience. Not only my own, but those of clients whom I've watched turn their health, and in many cases, *their lives,* around.

Back to your promise and mine: You promise to give me one month and I promise you'll wonder why you never exercised before. You will find yourself looking forward to exercising instead of dreading it, and hopefully spreading the word that movement can be natural, beneficial, and downright fun at any age.

Sal's Summary

In order for you to be able to see and feel these changes discussed here, it is critical to be persistent and challenge your body beyond what it is comfortable with or accustomed to handling in terms of variety of exercises and intensity. In return, you will quickly experience improvements in your quality of life. Over the longer term, you will also affect the quantity of your life. (Talk about getting two for the price of one.)

9

Details That Make the Difference

In order for strength training to be truly effective, it is vital to recognize there is more to being fit than just picking up a barbell or a pair of dumbbells and haphazardly moving them around in various directions. It takes careful thought, planning, and visualization. Once the importance of strength training is recognized, the next step is to approach it efficiently and safely. There are many factors to keep in mind when designing a strength-training program, particularly for older populations. As I mentioned in the overview, the three pillars needed to develop a successful exercise program are variety, proper technique, and intensity (a fourth, related pillar is proper nourishment). Here are the three exercise pillars for powerful, results-oriented workouts.

Variety

For long-term success, it is necessary for your body to be shocked on a regular basis—not with an electric current, but with new exercises. To prevent muscle adaptation (the point at which the body gets used to an exercise and stops progressing), you need to have a menu of exercise options for each muscle group. From that, you can select new options to replace the old ones every four to six weeks. A unique quality of this book is the array of exercise choices offered. It details a total of ninety-one strength exercises and twenty-two flexibility and balance exercises; this variety is the most conducive to long-term success. Never again need your body and mind get bored with exercise.

Proper Technique

As I tell each and every client, *"Technique is everything."* Without proper technique, you will not generate the results you desire and you will have a higher potential for injury. Technique is so essential that, for each exercise listed in Part Two, I provide the details needed for getting into position (another unique quality) *and* for actual execution of the movement. With each repetition you perform, always be mindful of technique.

In addition, there are four other variables to be aware of in order to ensure good form.

1. **Sequencing** of exercises is paramount to success. As important as it is, this one tends to get overlooked by many fitness books and fitness professionals. The basic rule of thumb here is that you should *always* work the larger muscles first, and the smaller muscles last. Larger muscles, such as the chest and back, rely on smaller muscles for support. For example, when you do a chest press, you are not only working your chest muscles, but also your shoulders and triceps. Chest muscles are the primary *muscle movers* while shoulders and triceps are the secondary *support muscles*. Because the chest relies on triceps for support, if triceps are pre-fatigued, they will interfere with your chest workout. Even within the realm of a given muscle group, some exercises recruit more muscle fibers than others. Therefore, when working out each individual muscle, the *large-to-smaller muscle* principle applies.

2. **Tempo** is the speed at which each repetition is performed. An ideal tempo is one that is moderate and slower on the negative than on the positive movement (in a rep, the negative movement is when the weight is being lowered). If you move too quickly, you will increase your chances for injury or will simply generate fewer positive results. The faster the movement, the fewer the number of muscle fibers activated to complete the action.

3. **Breathing** is the most basic and essential element of life. Yet, ironically, it tends to get overlooked frequently. As mundane as it may seem, breathing is critical for strength as well as overall health. There are basic breathing principles to help you generate better results and live with more zest. Here are some of them.

   - Always breathe *diaphragmatically.* In other words, instead of expanding the chest when inhaling, expand the abdominal region—this helps you take in more oxygen with each breath. When exhaling, compress your abs, forcing more air out of your lungs.

- When performing a resistance exercise, always exhale on exertion (the phase when resistance is being raised up against gravity—the positive movement). Inhale as a resistance is lowered—the negative movement. When you exhale, you have more power, and you need more strength during the *exertion* phase than during the *release* phase.

- Last but not least, always be sure to breathe. Never hold your breath. Breath-holding can place unnecessary stress on your heart, which can lead to fainting and even heart stoppage.

4. **Length** of strength workouts is important. Keep track of them and limit them to a range of forty-five to seventy-five minutes (beginners should start with a twenty-five to thirty-five minute range). Hormonal alterations and diminishing glycogen levels minimize the benefits of exercising longer than this. Additionally, as you become over-fatigued, you begin to overcompensate, sacrificing form, and thereby increasing your chances for injury.

Intensity

The key here is to avoid simply going through the motion. In order for the body to improve, it must be challenged beyond what it is accustomed to doing . . . even if the increments are slight. So as you become stronger, bump the intensity up a notch. This will not only prevent you from reaching a permanent plateau, which would ultimately contribute to degeneration, but will also keep you mentally stimulated. To vary the intensity, here are six variables you can play with (these are pertinent to those who have progressed beyond beginner levels).

1. **Loading.** This is the amount of resistance lifted. This one is obvious to most exercisers. The key is to bring your muscles to a state of fatigue. To do this effectively, you should sense fatigue, or feel a burn, by the last three to four repetitions of a given set. Please don't confuse this with the old saying, "No pain, no gain." This saying is just that: *old,* and dangerous. If you feel pain, then something's wrong. Either your technique is incorrect or the load is too heavy.

2. **Split routines.** This is a method of dividing your workouts so each one targets a different muscle group. This concept is covered extensively in Chapter 17, in the form of program options.

3. **Repetitions (reps).** The execution of a resistance movement, both upward and downward (positive and negative, respectively), one time. The number of reps to be performed for each set depends on what your goals are. Generally speaking, most people considering workouts relative to aging are primarily concerned with being leaner and maintaining, or improving, functionality. With that in mind, an ideal rep range is ten to twelve reps per set. The *more-reps-less-weight* concept is commonly known as the approach to follow. However, few people know exactly what *more reps* translates to and they choose weights that are so light, they'd be able to lift them fifteen, twenty, even 100 times. Always remember, doing more than twelve reps is going beyond the point of diminishing returns. When lifting a light weight too many times, there is not enough of a stimulus to generate strength gains. Instead, it becomes more a muscular endurance exercise and less a strengthening exercise.

4. **Set.** This represents one series of consecutive reps for one particular movement or exercise. An ideal number of sets is two per exercise for beginners, three sets for intermediate exercisers, and four sets for advanced.

5. **Frequency** of workouts per week is critical. You need to provide enough challenge to your body without overtraining it. Beginners should work out the whole body, with weights, twice per week. More experienced exercisers should work out three to four times per week performing split routines— challenging alternate muscle groups. The basic rule of thumb to adhere to is that the same muscle group should never be challenged two days in a row because muscles require forty-eight hours or more for recovery.

6. **Rest Interval** is a primary variable in attaining success, yet it is widely misunderstood or its effect is simply underestimated. How long you should rest depends on your goals and the intensity of your workout, but some rest is needed at three points in your workout.

   - *Between sets.* Most people reading this book are likely interested in being leaner and fully functioning, so rest intervals between sets should last between forty and fifty seconds.

   - *Between exercises or machines.* Although sixty seconds is preferable, try not to exceed ninety seconds.

   - *Between workouts.* Forty-eight hours is the ideal rest interval between workouts of a given muscle group—chest, shoulders, and triceps are considered one group, and back and biceps are considered the opposing muscle group. Be sure to avoid resting more than three days at a time.

Be in the Moment

Visualization of the primary muscles targeted is one more variable that helps with *proper technique* and *intensity* concurrently. This one makes a world of difference for each client, trainer, and acquaintance to whom I introduce it. A pet peeve of mine is when people get distracted while lifting weights. Some people chat with friends, others move to the beat of music or watch TV, some even read a book or magazine article. It's okay to chat while walking on a treadmill, or even read while exercising on a bike (although some research has shown the body burns fewer calories if you focus on other tasks when you're exercising). But when lifting weights, it's *not* okay to do or think of anything else but weightlifting. The mind is capable of contracting muscles on its own. If you're not focused, you could be contracting the wrong muscles (overstressing your neck or pulling on your lower back, for example) and not even know it.

If you're doing a set, and you catch yourself thinking about anything other than the actual performance of each and every rep—whether it's about your cranky boss, your delicious (healthful) post-workout meal, or your lovely spouse—end those thoughts immediately and replace them with a conscious focus on the muscle fibers of your target muscle group. The results will be amazing. Not only will you sense more power and strength (even using the same weights), but you will also develop a sense of oneness between your mind, body, and spirit. In other words, by focusing on nothing other than the rep you're performing, you may experience a meditative state. Be in the moment—always.

Part Two

Exercises:
Applications
and Illustrations

10

The How-To's of Exercise

art One of *Stop Aging—Start Training* lays out the foundation of health and fitness and covers the *why's* of exercise. Part Two is the *how-to's*. Accordingly, this second half of the book contains detailed exercise instructions, along with photographs and illustrations.

Machines versus Free Weights

Before discussing the actual exercises, there is one more source of confusion and debate I'd like to clear up, and that is whether machines or free weights are better. In a nutshell, neither is *better*. Both methods of resistance training have their advantages and their limitations. For that reason, I advocate using both in concert with each other. Although the most recent fitness trend has been to address functionality—the transfer of exercise benefits to everyday life—and therefore to lean away from machines and rely more on free weights, there still is a place for machine usage.

Machines are safer, particularly for the beginning exerciser or the older adult who may have experienced some strength losses, coupled with diminished balance and stability. Machines are an excellent way to build a strength foundation. Another advantage for machine usage is that, if well-designed, machines can more closely accommodate the *strength curve* for each muscle targeted. This pertains to the variability of a muscle's strength levels as you go through the range of motion in individual exercises. Free weights cannot accommodate this variability.

The disadvantage of relying solely on machines for strength gains is that they only challenge muscles in an isolated manner. Isolation of muscles is not ideal because the body does not function that way; its optimal functioning is through the recruitment of a synergy of muscles. Free weights can more closely mimic the basic functions of everyday life, and, thereby, can more easily transfer the benefits of training to day-to-day living. So, both styles of strength training are recommended.

Safety Suggestions

First and foremost, seek medical clearance, particularly if you fall into one of the following categories:

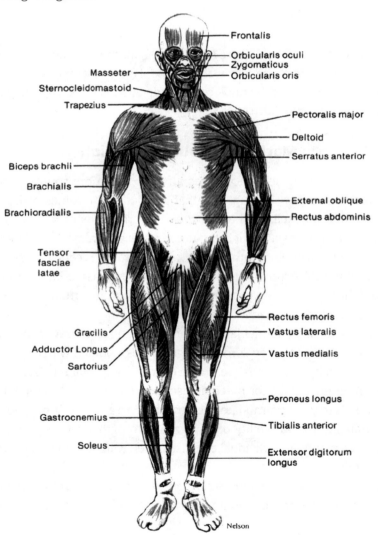

- You are a man over forty-five years of age
- You are a woman over fifty years of age
- You have a family history of heart disease or diabetes
- You have been sedentary for an extended period of time

For many of the exercises demonstrated, there are safety suggestions specific to each. In addition, there are several general safety factors that pertain to all exercises. They are as follows.

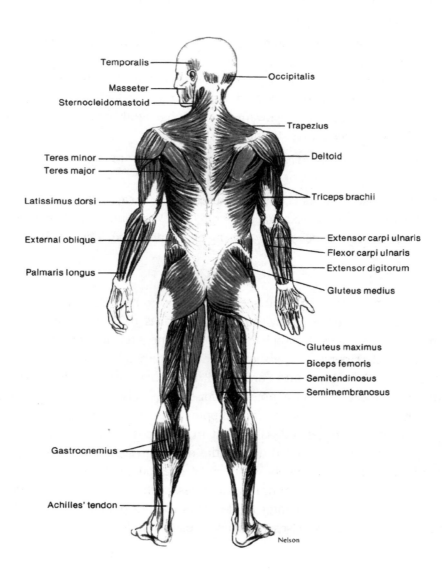

- Avoid locking out, or hyperextending, joints (this is when a joint is pushed past its normal range of motion). Always maintain a slight bend in the working joints at the end of each repetition.

- When performing exercises in a *supine* position (lying down, face up), keep the knees bent and positioned higher than the hips. This will prevent the back from hyperextending (bending too far backward), which places excess stress on the lower back.

- Prevent rapid, jerking movements. If you move too quickly, you will increase your chances for improper technique and you will not give the muscles enough of a challenge.

- Whether lying down, standing up, or sitting, always maintain a neutral spine. Avoid slouching over from the upper back and maintain the natural curve of the lower spine. If you're not sure what is the ideal neutral spine for the lower back, then, while standing flex your hips forward as much as possible and then extend backward (overarching). Settle into the position that is in between these two extremes.

- For upper body exercises, keep wrists in a neutral position. Prevent them from hyperextending or hyperflexing.

- Stay focused on your working muscles and always keep your neck and shoulder muscles relaxed (avoid shrugging). When unfocused, there is a tendency to overcompensate by tensing up the neck-shoulder region.

EXERCISES

Here are the exercises you've been waiting for. To help visualize the areas targeted for each exercise, view the figures on pages 100 and 101 illustrating the major muscle groups. A complete glossary of fitness terms begins on page 220.

These exercises were specifically selected for their effectiveness and safety and are broken down into compound (multi-joint) and simple (single-joint) movement sections. Please note that, for each exercise, I list the primary muscle movers followed by secondary, support muscles. For exercises that can be performed at home, as well as at the gym (no excuses allowed), an icon in the shape of a house is situated next to the name of the exercise. To exercise at home, some basic equipment will be needed, as outlined in Chapter 16.

Although I cover programming variables, such as exercise sequencing, in much greater detail in Chapter 17, it is helpful at this point to be mindful of the sequence in which exercises are listed for each muscle group.

11

Exercises— Lower Body

COMPOUND-MOVEMENT EXERCISES (MULTI-JOINT)

Squats

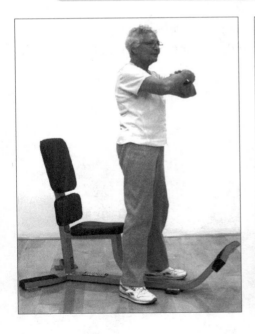 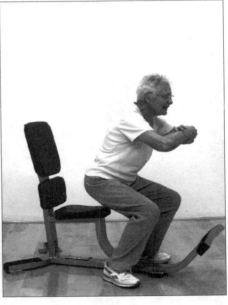

Muscles worked

- *Primary:* Quads (front thigh muscles), glutes (butt muscles), and hamstrings (rear thigh muscles).

- *Support:* Calf and shin (anterior tibialis).

Positioning

- Stand in front of a chair or bench, two feet away.

- Position feet parallel to each other, at hip-width distance.

- Maintain bend at the knees.

Movement

- While inhaling, slowly lower body, bending your knees and bringing your glutes back toward bench, as though you were going to sit.

- Lightly tap bench with glutes (or stop just before touching bench).

- As you exhale, slowly transition to the opposite direction, moving upward until you are fully standing again.

Helpful hints

- Prevent your knees from passing your toes.

- Keep your back as straight as possible.

- Use your abs for support and balance.

When you are able to perform 10–12 reps of this exercise easily, increase the intensity by performing squats without any support (chair or bench). As your strength and balance increase further, add resistance by carrying a dumbbell. Start with 5 pounds and build up from there.

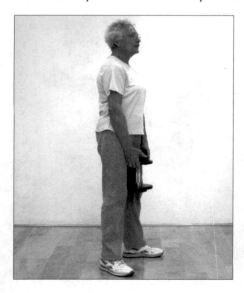
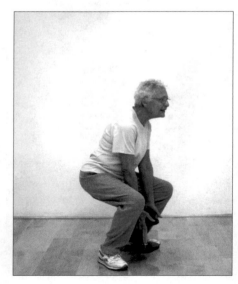

Lunges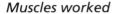

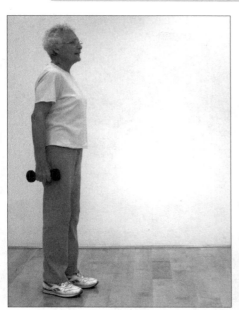
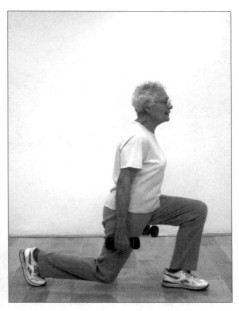

Muscles worked

• Primary: Quads, glutes, and hamstrings.

• Support: Calves and shins.

Positioning

• Hold weights in hands.

• Stand with feet parallel and four to six inches apart.

• Maintain slight bend at the knees.

• For first-timers, you may want to position yourself next to a bench or chair, so you can hold on for support if the need arises.

Movement

• While inhaling, step forward and slowly lower body, bending your knees while bringing your rear knee straight down toward floor.

• Stop descent when rear knee is one to two inches from floor.

• As you exhale, press your body back to the original position by extending your front leg (kick out).

• Alternate with other leg.

Helpful hints

• Prevent your front knee from passing your toes.

• Keep your back as straight as possible.

• Use your abs for support and balance.

Butt Press 🏠

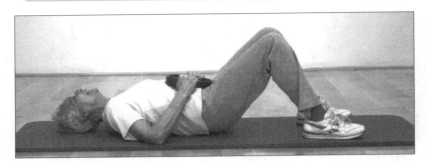

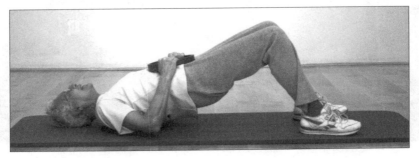

Muscles worked

- *Primary:* Glutes, quads, and hamstrings.
- *Support:* Abdominals.

Positioning

- Lie down on your back, face-up.
- Keep both knees bent, with feet flat on the floor.
- Hold a light to moderate-weight dumbbell or metal plate over your abdominals.

Movement

- While exhaling, press your hips upward, off the floor, as you contract your glutes.
- Press upward until your hips are in a straight line with your torso and thighs.
- As you inhale, slowly lower your hips toward the beginning position, stopping just before your glutes touch the floor.

Helpful hints

- Avoid hyper-extending (over-arching) your back when in the raised position.
- Be sure to squeeze your glutes together as you raise your hips.
- Use your abs for support.

(SINGLE-JOINT)

Seated Adduction

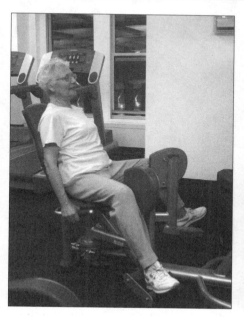 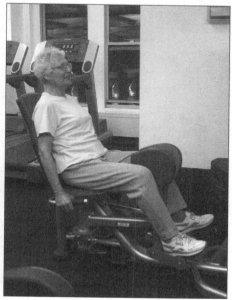

Muscles worked

• *Primary:* Adductors (inner thigh and groin muscles).

Positioning

• With leg cushions close together, sit on seat and place feet on pedals.

• Use hand lever to separate leg cushions as far as is comfortable.

• Lightly place hands on grips.

Movement

• As you exhale, press legs toward each other by contracting your adductors.

• Momentarily hold cushions together.

• As you inhale, slowly return your legs to the beginning position, stopping just before the plates touch.

Helpful hints

• Maintain firm abs for support.
• Avoid clasping hand grips too tightly.

Seated Abduction

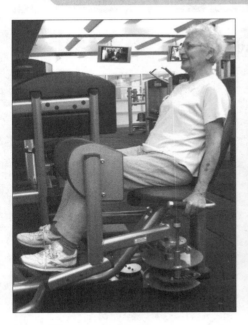 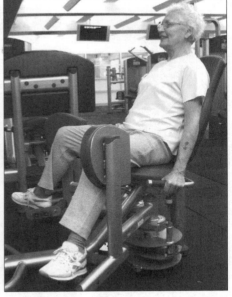

Muscles worked

• *Primary:* Abductors (outer thighs and glutes).

Positioning

• With leg cushions close together, sit on seat and place feet on pedals.

• Lightly place hands on grips.

Movement

• As you exhale, press legs outward by contracting your abductors and glutes.

• Continue pressing outward until you comfortably attain a full range of motion (ROM).

• Momentarily hold cushions in outermost position.

• As you inhale, slowly return your legs to the beginning position, stopping just before the plates touch.

Helpful hints

• Maintain firm abs for support.

• Avoid clasping hand grips too tightly.

Seated Leg Curl

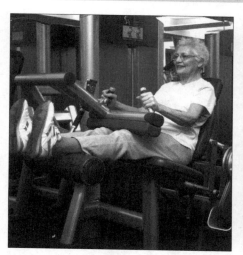 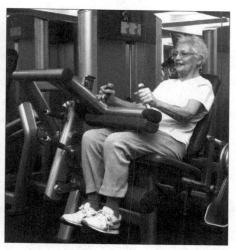

Muscles worked

- *Primary:* Hamstrings (backs of upper legs).
- *Support:* Calves and abs.

Positioning

- Adjust back cushion setting so knees are in alignment with machine's axis, while your back is fully supported by the cushion.
- Adjust leg cushion setting so cushion is positioned just above your Achilles tendons.
- Sit on seat and place legs on top of leg cushion.
- Lower thigh support onto thighs until legs are firmly supported (not squeezed tightly).
- Lightly place hands on grips.

Movement

- As you exhale, press legs downward by contracting your hamstrings.
- Continue pressing downward until you reach a ninety-degree angle at your knees.
- Momentarily hold weight.
- As you inhale, slowly raise your legs to the beginning position, stopping just before locking out your knees.

Helpful hints

- When in the uppermost position, avoid locking out knees.
- Avoid clasping hand grips too tightly.

Leg Extension

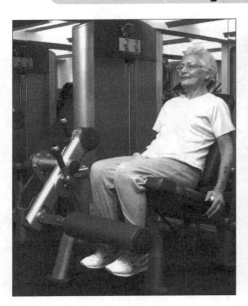 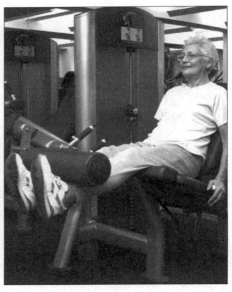

Muscles worked

• *Primary:* Quadriceps (quads—fronts of upper legs).

Positioning

• Adjust back cushion setting so knees are in alignment with machine's axis, while your back is fully supported by the cushion.

• Adjust ankle cushion setting so cushion is positioned just above your ankles.

• Sit on seat, place shins under leg cushion.

• Lightly place hands on grips.

Movement

• As you exhale, press legs upward by contracting your quads.

• Continue pressing upward until you fully extend your legs (just prior to locking out your knees).

• Momentarily hold weight.

• As you inhale, slowly lower your legs, stopping when your knees are at a ninety-degree angle.

Helpful hints

• When in the fully-extended position, avoid locking out knees.

• Avoid clasping hand grips too tightly.

Straight-Leg Calf Raise 🏠

There is also a seated variation of this exercise with straightened knees—not to be confused with the bent-knee seated calf raise (next exercise).

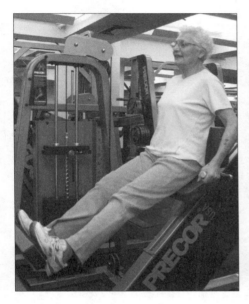 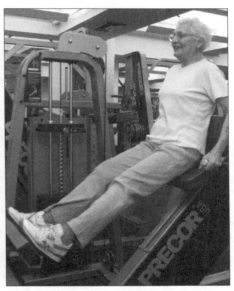

Muscles worked

• *Primary:* Gastrocnemius and soleus (outer and inner layers of calf muscle group, respectively).

• *Support:* Ankle and foot muscles.

Positioning

• Sit on seat, positioning hips against cushion.

• Straighten your legs, maintaining a slight bend at the knees.

Movement

• As you exhale, raise your heels by pressing into the balls of your feet, contracting your calf muscles.

• Press upward until you raise your heels as high as comfortably possible.

• Momentarily hold weight.

• As you inhale, slowly lower your heels, stopping when they are slightly below the level of your toes.

Here's a variation you can do with just a platform and a dumbbell.

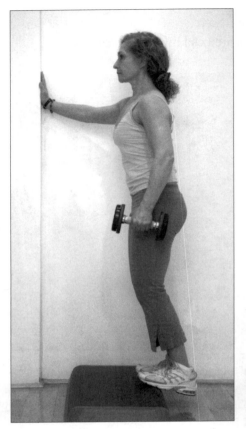 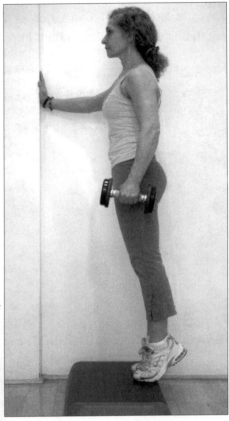

Helpful hints

• Throughout the ROM (range of motion), maintain a slight bend at your knees.

• Avoid dropping your heels too low below the toe level—this would potentially overstress your Achilles tendon.

Seated Calf Raise

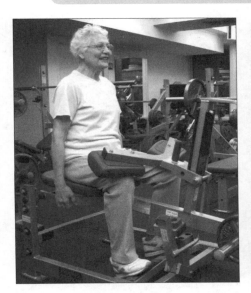 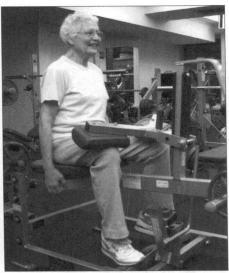

Muscles worked

• *Primary:* Soleus (inner layer of calf).

• *Support:* Ankle and foot muscles.

Positioning

• Place weight resistance on weight-holder.

• Adjust thigh cushion setting so your lower legs fit snuggly between platform and cushion.

• Remain seated upright.

• Position feet so the balls of your feet are on the platform, with your toes over the front edge.

• Hold grips gently.

Movement

• As you exhale, raise your heels by pressing into the balls of your feet, contracting your calf muscles.

• Press upward until you raise your heels as high as comfortably possible.

• Momentarily hold weight.

• As you inhale, slowly lower your heels, stopping when they are slightly below the level of your toes.

Helpful hints

• Avoid dropping your heels too low below the toe level—this would potentially overstress your Achilles tendon.

• Keep your knees positioned just past the cushion.

Anterior Tibialis Raise

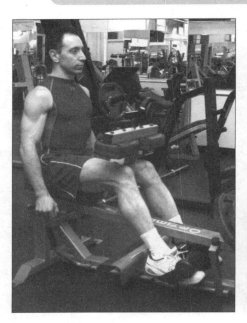
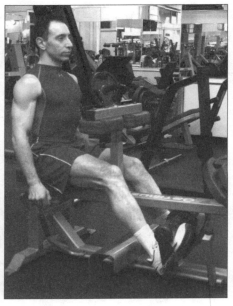

Muscles worked

- *Primary:* Anterior tibialis (anterior [front] muscles of the shin).
- *Support:* Ankle and foot muscles.

Positioning

- Place weight resistance on weight holder.
- Adjust thigh cushion high enough that your legs don't touch them during the exercise.
- Remain seated upright.
- Position feet onto foot pedals to allow for a pulling back motion.
- Hold grips gently.

Movement

- As you exhale, pull your toes upward, contracting your anterior tibialis.
- Raise your toes as high as comfortably possible.
- Momentarily hold weight.
- As you inhale, slowly lower your toes, stopping when you reach the beginning position.

Helpful hints

- For maximal results, avoid pressing your heels into the platform.
- When positioning yourself, slide your feet as far into the footstraps as possible and maintain that position throughout your set.

12

Exercises— Upper Body

CHEST

PRESSING EXERCISES

Standing Cable Decline Chest Press

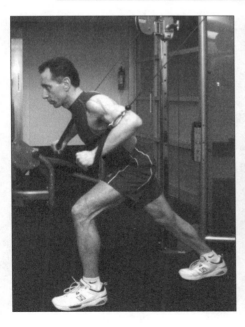 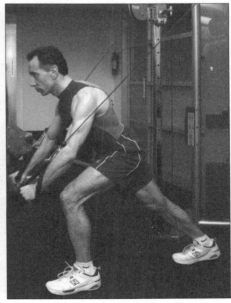

Muscles worked

• *Primary:* Lower to mid pectorals (chest muscles, also referred to as pecs).

• *Support:* Front deltoids (shoulders), triceps (rear upper arm), arm stabilizers and neutralizers, and core (abdominals, lower back).

Positioning

Using cable pulley system, with two closer pulleys than the traditional cable system (half as wide):

• Position grips so they are just below shoulder height.

• Stand in the center.

• Holding both grips, lunge forward so your body is angled forward (forty-five to sixty degrees).

• Position elbows at, or just past, your back, maintaining a forty-five-degree downward angle with your forearms.

Movement

• While exhaling, press downward at a forty-five-degree forward angle.

• Fully extend arms, stopping just before locking out your elbows.

• Inhale as you bring your elbows back.

• At all points throughout the range of motion (ROM), keep your elbows in alignment with your lower pecs.

Helpful hints

• Prevent your body from rocking forward and backward.

• On the return movement, prevent elbows from going too far past the back.

• Maintain firm abs for balance and to support your lower back.

• If you have shoulder sensitivity, lower the height of the grips.

Dumbbell Decline Chest Press

This is an advanced exercise. Be sure to have strong core muscles (abs and lower back) for support when getting on and off the bench.

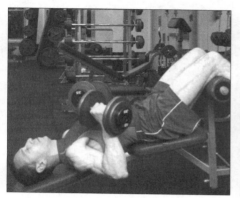 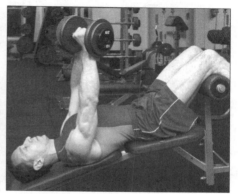

Muscles worked

• *Primary:* Lower to mid pectorals (pecs).

• *Support:* Front deltoids (delts), triceps, core (abdominals and lower back).

Positioning

• Place bench at a forty-forty-five degree decline angle (a bench with an elevated knee support is preferable).

• With a dumbbell in each hand, sit at the base of hump and place one leg at a time between cushions.

• Lie down, sliding dumbbells along legs to bring into position adjacent to lower pecs.

Movement

• While exhaling, contract your lower and mid pecs to press your arms upward.

• Move weights upward until your arms are fully extended.

• Pause briefly ($1/2$ second).

• While inhaling, slowly lower your arms to starting position.

Helpful hints

• Prevent your elbows from dropping lower than your back. If you go too low, your target muscles will rest too much while overstressing your shoulders (particularly rotator cuff muscles).

• Avoid benches that have an ankle support but no elevated knee pad. For the safety of your lower back, it is critical for your knees to be higher than your hips.

• Avoid locking out your elbows in the extended position.

Chest Press (Machine with Cables*)

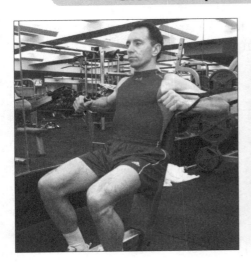
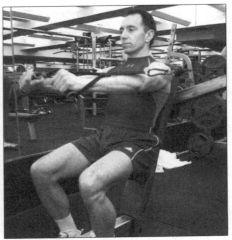

Muscles worked

• *Primary:* Mid pecs.

• *Support:* Some upper pecs, front delts, triceps, and arm stabilizers/neutralizers.

Positioning

• Place seat height so, when seated, the machine's cams (pulleys) will be adjacent to your rear shoulders.

• Reach for one grip at a time by turning your torso in the direction of that grip (if you reach for both grips simultaneously, you may overstress your shoulder [rear delt and/or rotator cuff] muscles).

• Place forearms at mid-pec level.

Movement

• While exhaling, contract from your pecs to press your arms forward and across in an arc-like motion.

• Stop just prior to locking out your elbows.

• After a brief pause, slowly return to the starting position, stopping when your forearms are adjacent to your pecs.

Helpful hints

• Maintain a ninety-degree angle at your knees. Placing your heels too far back (under your seat) will put extra stress on your lower back.

• Keep your elbows in alignment with your mid-pec region.

---

*Life Fitness or similar brands

Standing Cable Chest Press

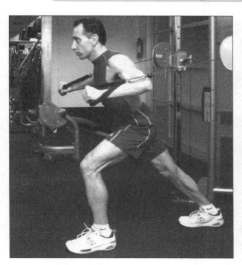 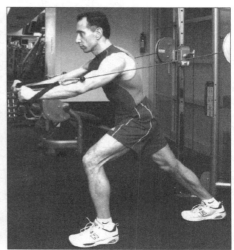

Muscles worked

- *Primary:* Mid pecs, arm stabilizers and neutralizers, and core (abs and lower back).
- *Support:* Some upper pecs, front delts, and triceps.

Positioning

Using the close-grip cable pulley system:

- Position grips so they are adjacent to mid and low pecs.
- Stand in the center.
- Hold both grips and lean forward slightly.
- Position elbows at, or just past, your back while positioning your forearms so they are perpendicular to your torso.

Movement

- While exhaling, press forward at a slightly downward angle, always keeping your arms perpendicular to your torso (at ninety degrees).
- Bring arms to a fully extended position, without locking out your elbows.
- Pause briefly.
- Inhale as you bring your elbows back to the starting position.
- At all points throughout the ROM, keep your elbows in alignment with your mid pecs.

Helpful hints

- Prevent your body from rocking forward and backward.
- On the return movement, prevent the elbows from going too far past the back.
- Maintain firm abs for support and balance.

Dumbbell Chest Press 🏠

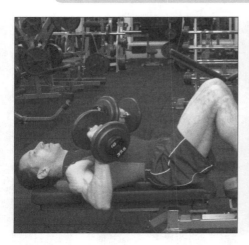
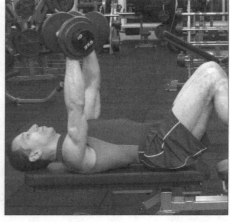

Muscles worked

- *Primary:* Mid pecs.

- *Support:* Some upper pecs, front delts, and triceps. Some abs will also be engaged.

Positioning

- Place bench at a flat, 180-degree angle.

- Sit on bench, placing dumbbells on thighs, just above knees.

- Lean back to lie on bench, while raising dumbbells into position using your legs.

- Bend knees and place feet on bench for back support.

- Position elbows at, or just past, back level.

- Position your forearms so they are perpendicular to your torso.

Movement

- While exhaling, contract your mid pecs to press your arms upward.

- Move arms upward until they are fully extended.

- Pause briefly.

- Slowly lower your arms to the starting position.

Helpful hints

- Prevent your elbows from dropping lower than your back (too low will allow too much rest for the target muscles, while overstressing the shoulders).

- Place your feet on the bench to support your lower back (always keep your knees higher than your hips).

- If you sense shoulder tightness, raise your head off the bench by two or so inches, as you lower the weights.

Ball Dumbbell Chest Press 🏠

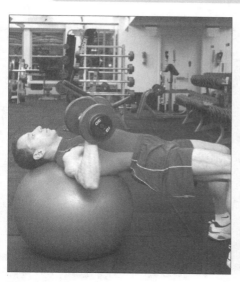 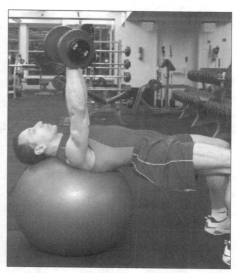

Muscles worked

- *Primary:* Mid pecs, arm stabilizers and neutralizers, and core (abs and lower back).
- *Support:* Some upper pecs, front delts, and triceps.

Positioning

- Sit on a stabilizer ball with dumbbells resting on thighs.
- Walk your feet forward, step by step, to roll downward, positioning your back on the ball while shifting the dumbbells to your chest.
- Continue to move forward so your head and shoulders rest on the ball.
- Keep your entire body in a straight horizontal line, preventing your hips from drooping downward.

Movement

- While exhaling, contract your mid pecs to help press your arms upward.
- Stop when your arms are fully extended.
- Pause briefly ($1/2$ second).
- While inhaling, slowly lower your arms to the starting position.

Helpful hints

- Prevent your elbows from dropping lower than your back.
- For more stability, keep your feet wider apart; as you improve in your strength and/or stability, bring your feet closer together.
- Avoid locking out your elbows in the extended position.

Dumbbell Incline Press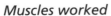

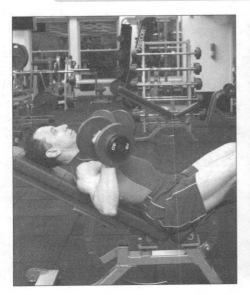
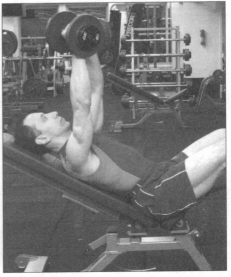

Muscles worked

- *Primary:* Upper pecs and front delts.
- *Support:* Triceps.

Positioning

- Position bench (seat and back portions) at a forty-five-degree angle.
- Sit on bench, placing dumbbells on thighs, just above knees.
- As you lean back into position, use your legs to raise dumbbells into position, with wrists adjacent to upper pecs.
- Place feet on a footrest (or stool) for back support.
- Position elbows at, or just past, your back level.
- Position your forearms so they are perpendicular to the floor.

Movement

- As you exhale, press arms upward, contracting primarily from your upper pecs.
- Press upward until your arms are fully extended.
- Pause briefly.
- While inhaling, slowly lower your arms to the starting position.

Helpful hints

- As you lower your arms, keep your elbows in alignment with upper pecs (not your shoulders).
- Prevent your elbows from moving past your back in the final downward position.
- Avoid locking out elbows.

CROSSOVER EXERCISES

Dumbbell Flyes

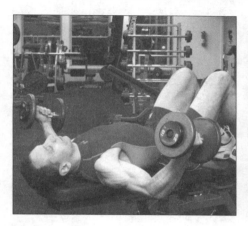 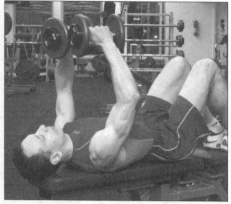

Muscles worked

- *Primary:* Outer pecs (outer ridge of chest muscles) and front delts.
- *Support:* Triceps.

Positioning

- Place bench at a flat, 180-degree angle.
- Sit on bench, placing dumbbells on thighs, just above knees.
- Lean back to lie on bench, while raising dumbbells into position using your legs.
- Bend knees and place feet on bench for back support.
- Raise dumbbells so they are held over your chest, with elbows pointed outward in a slightly bent position.

Movement

- While inhaling, lower weights out to the sides, maintaining a slight bend at elbows.
- Stop when your elbows are adjacent to the bottom of your back—or sooner, if you begin to feel pulling on your shoulders.
- As you exhale, press arms upward, contracting primarily from your outer pecs (this movement resembles hugging a tree).

Helpful hints

- As you lower your arms, keep your elbows in alignment with mid pecs (not your shoulders).
- Prevent your elbows from moving past your back in the final downward position
- Maintain a fixed open angle at your elbows throughout the ROM.

Cable Crossover

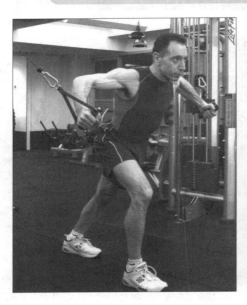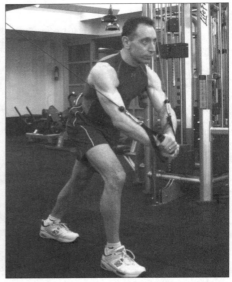

Muscles worked

- *Primary:* Outer pecs (outer ridge of chest muscles) and front delts.
- *Support:* Triceps.

Positioning

Using the wide-pulley (traditional) cable pulley system:

- Stand in the center.
- Hold grips and lean forward slightly.
- Position elbows at, or just past, your back while positioning your forearms so they are sloped downward toward floor.

Movement

- While exhaling, contract your outer pecs as you press your arms across your chest toward each other, maintaining a slight bend at elbows (this movement resembles hugging a tree).
- Overlap hands in front of you.
- Hold momentarily.
- As you inhale, lower the weights by allowing arms to return to beginning position—open arms.

Helpful hints

- Throughout your ROM, keep your elbows in alignment with mid pecs (not your shoulders).
- Prevent your elbows from moving too far past your back in the upward position.
- Maintain a fixed open angle at your elbows.

BACK

PULLDOWN EXERCISES

Latissimus Dorsi (Lat) Pulldown—Standard (Straight) Bar

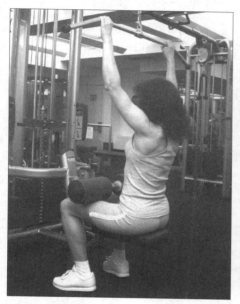

Muscles worked

- *Primary:* Lats and rhomboids.
- *Support:* Biceps, rear delts, and forearms.

Positioning

- Position seat height, or pad height (depending on machine design), so thighs are secured under cushion.

- Stand up to hold bar, keeping hands in such a position that, as you pull the bar downward, your elbows will be at ninety-degrees when your biceps (upper arms) are parallel to the floor.

- Keep back straight, maintaining shoulders over hips.

- Arc from your mid torso, from your sternum (chest bone)—as opposed to leaning back from the hips.

Movement

- While exhaling, contract your lats, pulling your elbows down toward the sides of your torso.

- Stop when the bar is just below your chin (going too low will stress your rotator cuff).

- As you inhale, use your lats to slowly lower the weights, raising your arms to a fully extended position, stopping just before locking out your elbows.

Helpful hints

- Prevent your torso from rocking.

- Avoid tilting your forearms forward as you pull downward— keep your elbows in alignment with your wrists.

- Avoid tightening up your neck and shoulders (no shoulder shrugs).

Lat Pulldown—Straps (Bilateral)

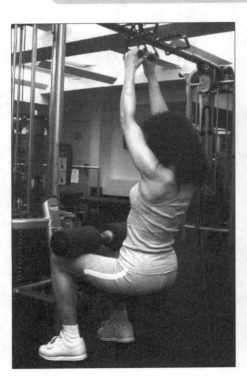 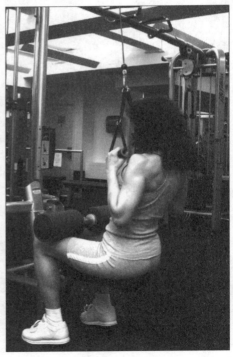

Muscles worked

- *Primary:* Lats and rhomboids.
- *Support:* Biceps, rear delts, and forearms.

Positioning

- Position seat height, or pad height (whichever is adjustable), so thighs are secured under cushion.
- Hold hand straps with palms facing one another..
- Keep back straight, maintaining shoulders over hips.
- Arc from your mid torso—your sternum—as opposed to leaning back from the hips.

Movement

- While exhaling, contract your lats, pulling your elbows down toward the sides of your torso.
- Stop when your wrists are just above shoulder height.
- As you inhale, slowly lower the weights, raising your arms to a fully extended position, stopping just before locking out your elbows.
- At all points throughout the ROM, keep your elbows in alignment with your wrists.

Helpful hints

- Prevent your torso from rocking forward and backward.
- As you pull downward, keep your elbows slightly ahead of your torso, as opposed to pulling them back too far.

Standing Rope Pulldown

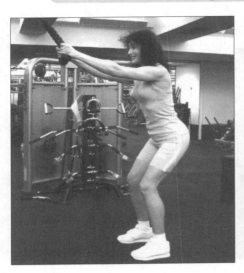 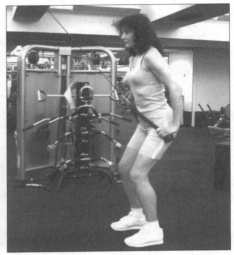

Muscles worked

• *Primary:* Lats, traps (trapezius), rhomboids, and serratus anterior (riblike muscles under the pecs).

• *Support:* Biceps, rear delts, triceps, and abs.

Positioning

• Attach rope to a high pulley.

• Stand with feet hip-width apart.

• Maintain slight bend at knees and hips (thirty-five to forty-five degrees at both joints).

• Lean forward slightly.

• Arc lower back while maintaining firm abs.

• Hold rope ends with both hands.

• Maintain slight bend at elbows.

Movement

• While exhaling, contract your lats downward and toward each other, pulling your elbows down toward the sides of your torso.

• Stop when your hands reach just outside your thighs.

• As you inhale, slowly allow the weights to bring your arms to the beginning position, stopping when your hands are at nose level.

Helpful hints

• Prevent your elbows from locking out or changing angles—if you flex and extend at the elbows, you will work more of your triceps and less of your back.

• Avoid gripping the rope too tightly.

• Be sure to keep your knees and toes in alignment.

Dumbbell Pullover 🏠

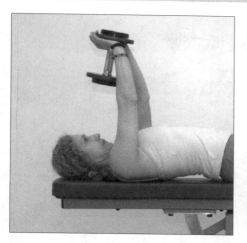
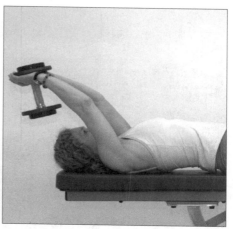

Muscles worked

- *Primary:* Lats, traps (trapezius), rhomboids, and serratus anterior.
- *Support:* Pecs, biceps, rear delts, triceps, and abs.

Positioning

- Place bench at a flat, 180-degree angle.
- Sit on bench, placing dumbbell on one thigh, just above knee.
- Lean back to lie on bench, while raising dumbbell into position using your leg.
- Bend knees and place feet on bench for back support.
- Hold dumbbell with both hands directly over chin, maintaining a slight bend at elbows.
- Position your forearms so they are parallel to each other, with elbows pointed at knees.

Movement

- While inhaling, lower dumbbell backward, bringing it just past your head.
- Stop just before you sense tightness in your shoulders.
- Pause momentarily.
- As you exhale, contract your back muscles as you slowly raise the weight to the beginning position, stopping when the dumbbell is over your chin again.

Helpful hints

- Prevent your elbows from locking out or changing angles—if you flex and extend at the elbows, you will work more of your triceps and less of your back.
- Avoid gripping the dumbbell too tightly.
- Be sure to keep your knees and toes in alignment.

ROW EXERCISES

Cable One-Arm Row

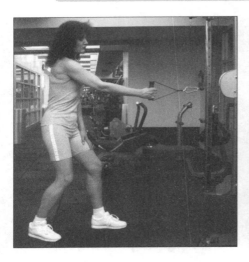 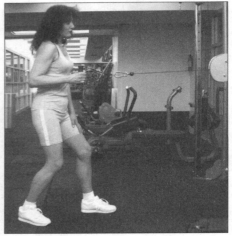

Muscles worked

- *Primary:* Lats, traps, and rhomboids.
- *Support:* Biceps, rear delts, and abs.

Positioning

- Attach handle to a mid-range pulley.
- Stand with feet hip-width apart and one foot forward (opposite from working arm).
- Maintain slight bend at knees (thirty-five to forty-five degrees at both joints).
- Maintain straight posture (shoulders over hips).
- Step back, away from weight rack, to allow for full ROM of the working arm.

Movement

- As you exhale, contract your working lat (squeezing your shoulder blade), moving it toward the resting lat, bringing your elbow straight back.
- Keep your elbow close to your torso as you move through the ROM.
- Stop when your elbow passes your back by one or two inches.
- As you inhale, slowly extend your arm forward to the beginning position, as you lower the weights.

Helpful hints

- Prevent your elbow from locking out when in the extended position.
- Lightly cup your hand around the handle; avoid gripping tightly.
- Keep your knees and toes in alignment.

Dumbbell One-Arm Row

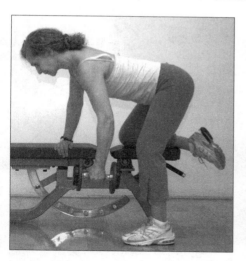
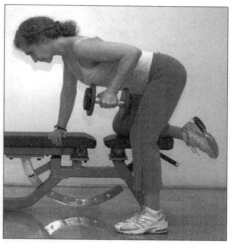

Muscles worked

- *Primary:* Lats, traps, and rhomboids.
- *Support:* Biceps, rear delts, and abs.

Positioning

- Place your dumbbell on the floor next to the center of the bench.
- Place bench at a flat, 180-degree angle.
- Position the knee and hand of non-working side onto bench (to protect your wrist, turn your hand inward so your fingers hang over the edge of the bench toward your midline).
- Place the foot of your working side on the floor out to your side so that both knees and both hips are parallel.
- Maintain a flat back, keeping both shoulder blades parallel.

Movement

- As you exhale, contract your working lat (squeezing your shoulder blade), moving it toward the resting lat, bringing your elbow straight back.
- Keep your elbow close to your torso as you move through the ROM.
- Stop when your elbow passes your back by one or two inches.
- As you inhale, slowly extend your arm forward to the beginning position, as you lower the dumbbell.

Helpful hints

- Prevent your elbow from locking out when in the extended position.
- Lightly cup your hand around the handle.
- Be sure to keep your knees and toes in alignment.

Seated (Machine) Row

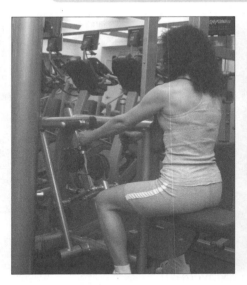 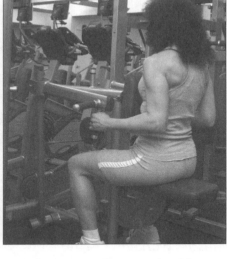

Muscles worked

- *Primary:* Lats, traps, and rhomboids.
- *Support:* Biceps and rear delts.

Positioning

- Position seat height so when you hold grips while seated, your shoulders are higher than your wrists by three or four inches.
- Position chest cushion so you are not forced to overreach, yet are capable of performing a full ROM.
- Arc upper torso slightly away from chest cushion.
- Keep chin level (avoid looking up or down).

Movement

- As you exhale, contract your lats together, squeezing your shoulder blades toward each other.
- Keep your elbows close to your torso as you move through the ROM.
- Stop when your elbows pass your back by one or two inches.
- As you inhale, slowly extend your arms forward to the beginning position, as you lower the weights.

Helpful hints

- Avoid leaning back, away from the cushion, as you pull the weights.
- Lightly cup your hands around the handles—avoid clasping.
- Avoid overreaching, forcing your shoulders to roll forward.
- Be sure to keep your knees and toes in alignment.

Standing (Cable) Low Row

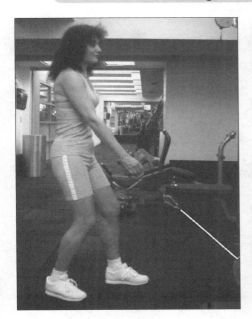
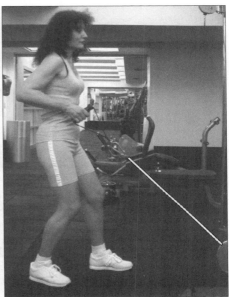

Muscles worked

• *Primary:* Upper lats, mid and upper traps, and rhomboids.

• *Support:* Biceps and rear delts.

Positioning

• Attach handle to a low pulley.

• Stand with feet hip-width apart and one foot forward (opposite from working arm).

• Maintain slight bend at knees (thirty-five to forty-five degrees).

• Maintain straight posture (shoulders over hips).

• Step back, away from weights, to allow for full ROM of the working arm.

Movement

• As you exhale, contract your working lat (squeezing your shoulder blade), moving it toward the resting lat, bringing your elbow up and back.

• Keep your elbow close to your torso as you move through the ROM.

• Stop when your elbow passes your back by one or two inches.

• As you inhale, slowly extend your arm forward to the beginning position, as you lower the resistance.

Helpful hints

• Prevent your elbow from locking out when in the extended position.

• Lightly cup your hand around the handle; avoid gripping tightly.

ROTATOR CUFF EXERCISES

Dumbbell External Rotation

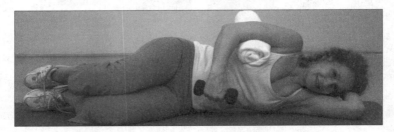

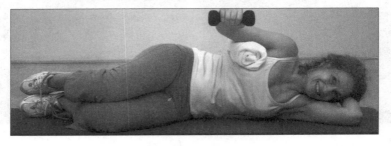

Muscles worked

- *Primary:* External rotators of the shoulder joint.
- *Support:* Abs and forearms.

Positioning

- Place a rolled-up towel under your working arm.
- With a light weight in your working hand, lie down on your non-working side (on a bench or exercise mat).
- Maintain a forty-five-degree bend at knees.
- Rest your head on your lower forearm.
- Maintain straight posture (prevent your waistline from drooping down or your head from being pressed up).

Movement

- As you exhale, move your working hand upward, always maintaining a ninety-degree angle at your elbow.
- Move weight upward until your hand/forearm is slightly higher than a horizontal position.
- As you inhale, slowly return your hand/forearm to the beginning position, as you lower the resistance.
- Stop just before your hand (or weight) touches your torso.

Helpful hints

- Maintain firm abs throughout the ROM.
- Keep your body tilted slightly forward (ten to fifteen degrees).

Cable External Rotation

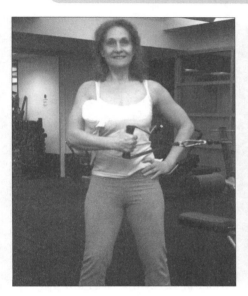 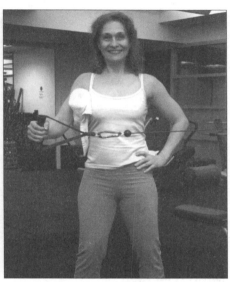

Muscles worked

- *Primary:* External rotators of the shoulder joint.
- *Support:* Abs and forearms.

Positioning

- Attach handle to a mid-range pulley.
- Place a rolled-up towel under your working arm.
- Stand with feet hip-width apart and with body perpendicular to cable pulley (the working side is further from the machine).
- Maintain slight bend at knees (thirty-five to forty-five degrees).
- Sidestep, away from weight stack, to allow for full ROM of the working arm.
- Maintain straight posture (shoulders over hips).

Movement

- As you exhale, rotate your working arm outward, maintaining a ninety-degree angle at your elbow.
- Move outward until your hand is just past the position of your elbow.
- As you inhale, slowly return your hand/forearm to the beginning position, lowering the resistance.

Helpful hints

- Maintain firm abs throughout the ROM.
- Avoid shifting your weight from your resting side to your working side as you go through the ROM.

Cable Internal Rotation

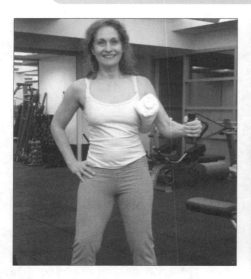 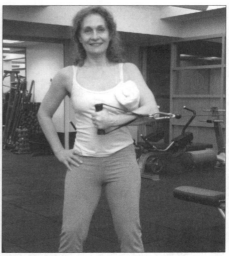

Muscles worked

- *Primary:* Internal rotators of the shoulder joint.
- *Support:* Abs and forearms.

Positioning

- Attach handle to a mid-range pulley.
- Place a rolled-up towel under your working arm.
- Stand with feet hip-width apart and with body perpendicular to cable pulley (the working side is closer to the machine).
- Maintain slight bend at knees (thirty-five to forty-five degrees).
- Maintain straight posture (shoulders over hips).
- Sidestep, away from weights, to allow for full ROM for the working arm.
- Bring working hand to a slightly wider angle than your elbow by ten to twenty degrees.

Movement

- As you exhale, move your working hand inward, toward your abs, always maintaining a ninety-degree angle at your elbow.
- Move inward until your hand lightly presses against your abs.
- As you inhale, slowly return your hand to the beginning position.

Helpful hints

- Maintain firm abs throughout the ROM.
- Avoid shifting your weight from your working side to your resting side as you go through the ROM.
- Always keep your neck and shoulder region relaxed.

DELTOID EXERCISES

Dumbbell Rear Deltoid 🏠

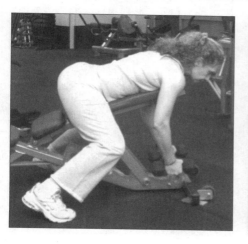 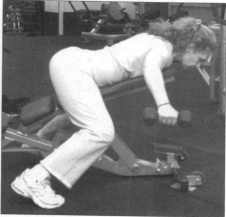

Muscles worked

- *Primary:* Rear delts and mid traps.
- *Support:* Upper lats and upper traps.

Positioning

- Position bench at a slight incline angle (twenty-five to thirty degrees).
- Position dumbbells below head of bench.
- Lie face-down on bench, positioning chin beyond edge of bench.
- Straddle bench, placing feet on the floor, on each side of bench.
- Have palms face each other, while pointing elbows outward to the sides.

Movement

- While exhaling, raise your arms outward to the sides, maintaining a slight bend at your elbows.
- Move upward until your elbows are adjacent to your back.
- As you inhale, slowly lower the weights, returning your arms to the beginning position.
- At the bottom position, stop just prior to the point at which your wrists are directly under your shoulders.

Helpful hints

- Maintain firm abs throughout the ROM.
- Keep your neck and shoulder region relaxed.
- Avoid the temptation to bend your elbows as you raise your arms.

Standing (Cable) Rear Deltoid

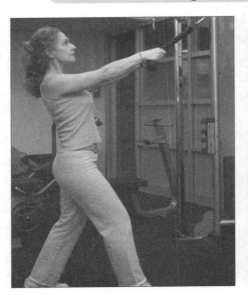 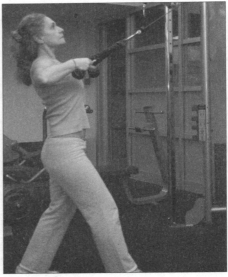

Muscles worked

- *Primary:* Rear delts and traps.
- *Support:* Abs, upper lats, and back extensors.

Positioning

- Position pulley at a high setting.
- Hold on to strap grips or rope.
- Step three to five feet back from machine.
- Maintain an open stance, with one foot slightly ahead of the other and feet hip-width apart.
- Lean back slightly.
- Have palms face each other, while pointing elbows outward to sides.

Movement

- As you exhale, contract your rear delts towards your spine, moving your elbows straight back.
- Keep your elbows elevated at shoulder level.
- Stop when your elbows pass your back by one or two inches.
- As you inhale, extend your arms forward to the beginning position, slowly lowering the weights.

Helpful hints

- Prevent your elbows from locking out when in the extended position.
- Lightly cup your hands around the handle.
- Be sure to keep your knees and toes in alignment.
- Maintain firm abs throughout the ROM.

(Machine) Rear Deltoid

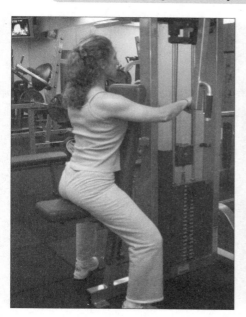
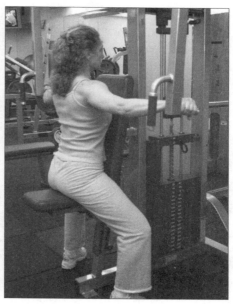

Muscles worked

- *Primary:* Rear delts and mid traps.
- *Support:* Upper lats and upper traps.

Positioning

- Position seat at a height that would allow your hands to be just below shoulder height (two to three inches)
- Rest chest against cushion and maintain a slight arc at your lower back.
- While holding grips, maintain a slight bend at your elbows.

Movement

- As you exhale, move your arms outward, to the sides, and back, squeezing from your rear delts.
- Move arms back until your elbows are either one to two inches beyond your back or adjacent to your back, depending on flexibility.
- As you inhale, slowly lower the weights, returning your arms to the beginning position.
- Stop just prior to the point where the weights touch.

Helpful hints

- Initiate from your rear delts, not from your arm muscles.
- Avoid the temptation to bend your elbows as you move your arms back.

Dumbbell Shoulder Press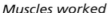

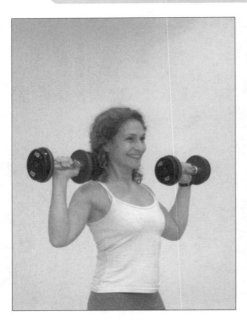 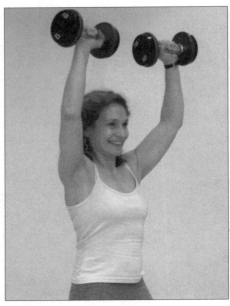

Muscles worked

- *Primary:* Delts—front, medial, and rear.
- *Support:* Abs and traps.

Positioning

- Hold dumbbells in hands.
- Stand with feet hip-width apart and with a slight bend at your knees (twenty-five to thirty degrees).
- Maintain straight posture (shoulders over hips, and hips over ankles).
- Position your arms so your wrists are adjacent to your shoulders.

Movement

- As you exhale, press the weights

upward, extending your arms from the elbows.

- Move upward until your elbows are almost straight (stop just before locking them out).
- Slowly lower the weights, bringing your arms to the beginning position, with wrists at shoulder height.

Helpful hints

- Maintain firm abs throughout the ROM
- Always keep your wrists situated over elbows.
- Maintain a slight bend at your knees.

Anterior Deltoids (Cable)

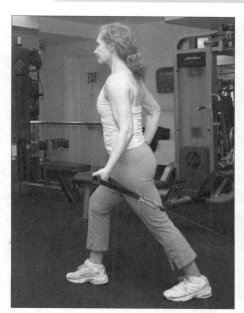 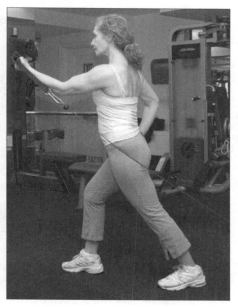

Muscles worked

- *Primary:* Anterior (front) delts.
- *Support:* Biceps, abs, and forearms.

Positioning

- Position pulley at a low setting.
- Hold on to a strap grip.
- Step forward three to five feet away from machine.
- Maintain an open stance, with one foot (from the non-working side) ahead of the other and feet hip-width apart.
- Maintain an upright posture.

Movement

- As you exhale, press the resistance upward, extending your arm forward.
- Move upward until your biceps (upper arm) are parallel to the floor.
- Slowly lower the resistance, bringing your arm to the beginning position, adjacent to your torso.

Helpful hints

- Maintain firm abs throughout the ROM.
- Keep your wrists straight throughout the ROM.
- Maintain a slight bend at your elbow and knees.

Anterior Deltoids (Dumbbells)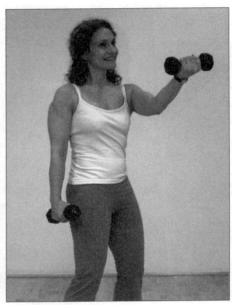

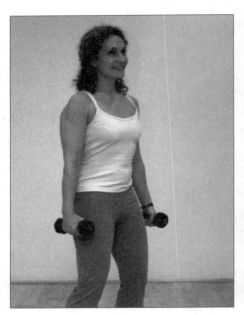

You can also do this exercise with dumbbells.

- Keep your feet parallel while maintaining a slight bend at your knees.
- Begin with your arms to your sides and palms facing your legs.
- Raise arms in an alternating fashion—as you raise the working arm, slowly turn your palm upward.
- As you lower one arm, begin raising the alternate.

ARMS

BICEPS—FRONT UPPER ARMS

Preacher Bench Curls (E-Z Bar or Dumbbells)

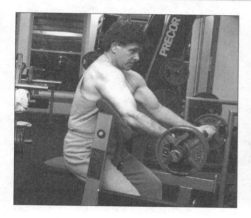 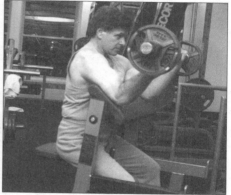

Muscles worked

- *Primary:* Biceps (main frontal area).
- *Support:* Forearms, front delts.

Positioning

- Position seat at a height that would allow you to rest your upper arms (triceps) on the cushion (if the seat is too high, you will put pressure on your elbows; if the seat is too low, you will stress your neck and shoulders).

- Straddle seat as you reach for the barbell (E-Z grip).

- With barbell in hands, seat yourself and avoid locking out your elbows (rest chest against cushion).

Movement

- As you exhale, curl your arms upward, lifting barbell toward your shoulders.

- Stop prior to having your wrists directly over your elbows (prevent your forearms from reaching a position that's perpendicular to the floor).

- As you inhale, slowly lower the barbell, returning your arms to the beginning position.

- Stop just prior to locking out your elbows.

Helpful hints

- Avoid shrugging (tightening) your neck and shoulders.

- If you prefer using dumbbells, everything is the same; keep palms slightly turned toward each other.

Concentrated Curls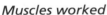

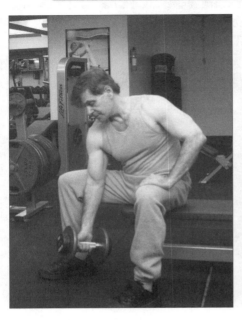 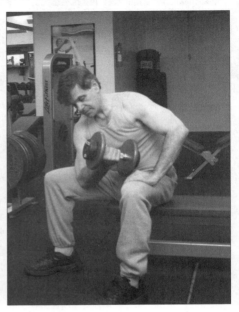

Muscles worked

- *Primary:* Biceps (main).
- *Support:* Forearms.

Positioning

- Sit on the edge of a bench or seat.
- Position your non-working hand on your adjacent thigh for back support.
- Rest the triceps of your working arm against the inside of your other leg—1 to 2 inches from the knee.
- Position the elbow just below the bottom of your thigh.

Movement

- Curl your working arm upward, lifting dumbbell toward your opposite shoulder, while exhaling.

- Raise weight as high as possible—until the weight touches your chest or until you reach a full ROM.
- Hold contraction for $1/2$ second.
- As you inhale, slowly lower the dumbbell, returning your arm to the beginning position.
- Stop just prior to locking out your elbow.

Helpful hints

- During the upward movement, avoid bringing weight outward—instead, move weight directly toward opposite shoulder, in a straight line across your torso.
- Avoid shrugging (tightening) your neck and shoulders.

Standing Curl Twists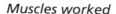

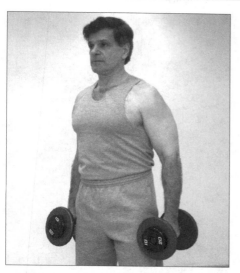
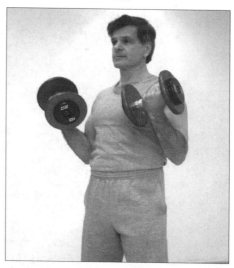

Muscles worked

• *Primary:* Biceps (main frontal and outer areas).

• *Support:* Forearms and abs.

Positioning

• Hold dumbbells in hands.

• Stand with feet hip-width apart and a slight bend at your knees.

• Maintain straight posture (shoulders over hips, and hips over ankles).

• Position your arms at the sides of your body, with a slight bend at the elbows.

Movement

• As you exhale, curl your arms upward, moving the weights as far as you can without shifting elbows forward.

• As you lift the weights, gradually twist forearms, turning palms upward (in the final position, palms should face your shoulders).

• Hold contraction for $1/2$ second.

• Slowly lower the weights, returning your arms to the straightened, but unlocked, position.

• While lowering the weights, gradually turn palms inward (in the final position, palms should face your outer thighs).

Helpful hints

• Maintain firm abs throughout the ROM.

• Avoid leaning back as you raise the weights.

• Avoid leaning forward as you lower the weights.

Cable Curls (with E-Z Grip)

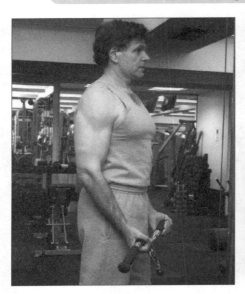 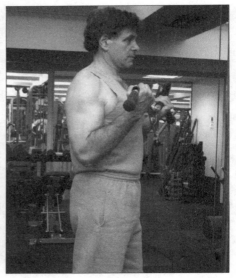

Muscles worked

- *Primary:* Biceps (main).
- *Support:* Forearms, abs, and back.

Positioning

- Hold grip in hands, palms up.
- Stand close to a low pulley, with feet hip-width apart and a slight bend at your knees.
- Maintain a straight posture (shoulders over hips, and hips over ankles).
- Position your arms at sides of your body, with only a slight bend at the elbows.

Movement

- As you exhale, curl your arms upward.

- Move weights upward until attaining a full ROM (keep elbows to your sides, avoid shifting elbows forward).
- Hold contraction for $1/2$ second.
- Slowly lower the weights, bringing your arms to the straightened, but unlocked, position.

Helpful hints

- Maintain firm abs throughout the ROM.
- Avoid leaning back as you raise the weights.
- Avoid leaning forward as you lower the weights.

Hammer Curl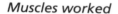

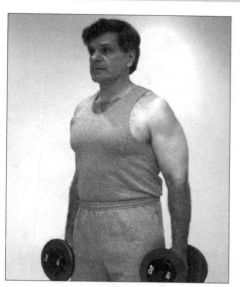
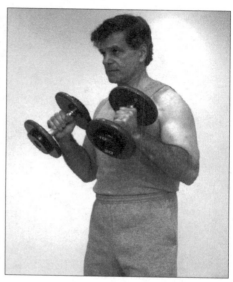

Muscles worked

- *Primary:* Biceps (outer, lateral area).
- *Support:* Forearms and abs.

Positioning

- Hold dumbbells in hands.
- Stand with feet hip-width apart and a slight bend at your knees.
- Maintain straight posture (shoulders over hips, and hips over ankles).
- Position your arms at sides of your body, with only a slight bend at the elbows.

Movement

- As you exhale, curl your arms upward, moving weights until attaining a full ROM (keep elbows to your sides—avoid shifting them forward).
- Hold contraction briefly.
- Slowly lower the weights, while inhaling, bringing your arms to the straightened, but unlocked, position.

Helpful hints

- Maintain firm abs.
- Keep your wrists straight throughout the ROM.
- Avoid leaning back as you raise the weights.
- Avoid leaning forward as you lower the weights.

Rope Hammer Curls

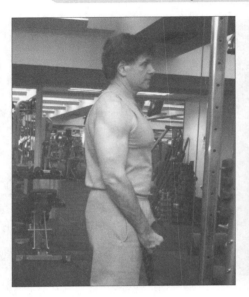
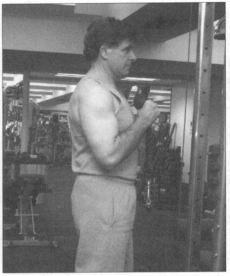

Muscles worked

- *Primary:* Biceps (outer, lateral area).
- *Support:* Forearms and abs.

Positioning

- Position rope grip at lowest pulley angle.
- Hold ends of the rope.
- Stand with feet hip-width apart and one foot forward (maintain a slight bend at your knees).
- Maintain straight posture (shoulders over hips, and hips over ankles).
- Position your arms at the sides of your body, with a slight bend at the elbows.

Movement

- As you exhale, curl your arms upward, moving the weights until attaining a full ROM (keep elbows to your sides—avoid shifting elbows forward).
- Hold contraction for $1/2$ second.
- Slowly lower the weights, while inhaling, bringing your arms to the beginning position.

Helpful hints

- Maintain firm abs.
- Keep your wrists straight throughout the ROM.
- Avoid leaning back as you raise the weights.
- Avoid leaning forward as you lower the weights.

TRICEPS (REAR UPPER ARMS)

Although the following three exercises look similar and are done on the same machine, they target different areas of the triceps due to the use of different grips.

E-Z Grip Cable Triceps Pressdown

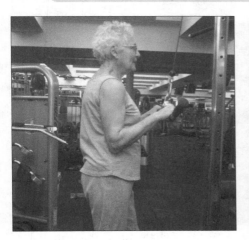 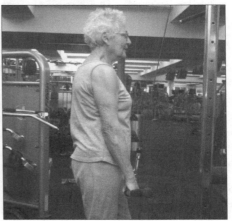

Muscles worked

- *Primary:* Triceps (all three heads).
- *Support:* Abs and shoulders.

Positioning

- Position E-Z grip at high pulley.
- Hold grip with hands pronated (face down).
- Stand with feet hip-width apart and one foot forward (maintain a slight bend at your knees).
- Maintain straight posture (shoulders over hips, and hips over ankles).
- Hold abs firmly.
- Position your elbows at the sides of your body, with hands at chest level.

Movement

- As you exhale, press the grip downward until your arms are straight, but unlocked (keep elbows to your sides throughout the ROM).
- Hold the contraction $\frac{1}{2}$ second.
- Slowly raise your forearms, while inhaling, bringing your hands to a chest-level position.

Helpful hints

- Maintain firm abs.
- Always keep your neck and shoulders relaxed.
- Avoid leaning forward as you press down.
- Keep your wrists straight.

V Grip Cable Triceps Pressdown

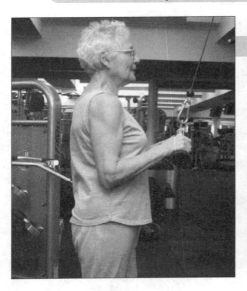 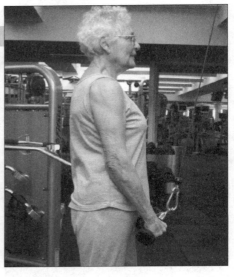

Muscles worked

- *Primary:* Mid and outer portions of triceps.
- *Support:* Abs and shoulders.

Positioning

- Position V grip at high pulley.
- Hold grip with hands pronated (face down).
- Stand with feet hip-width apart and one foot forward (maintain a slight bend at your knees).
- Maintain straight posture (shoulders over hips, and hips over ankles).
- Position your elbows at the sides of your body, with hands at chest level.

Movement

- As you exhale, press the grip downward until your arms are straight, but unlocked (keep elbows to your sides throughout the ROM).
- Hold contraction for $1/2$ second.
- Slowly raise your forearms, while inhaling, bringing your hands to a chest-level position.

Helpful hints

- Maintain firm abs.
- Always keep your neck and shoulders relaxed.
- Avoid leaning forward as you press down.
- Keep your wrists straight.

Rope Triceps Pressdown

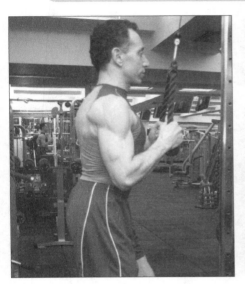 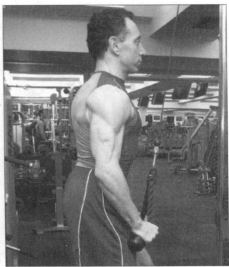

Muscles worked

- *Primary:* Outermost, lateral portion of triceps.
- *Support:* Abs and shoulders.

Positioning

- Position rope grip at high pulley.
- Hold ends of the rope.
- Stand with feet hip-width apart and one foot forward (maintain a slight bend at your knees).
- Maintain straight posture (shoulders over hips, and hips over ankles).
- Position your elbows at the sides of your body, with hands at chest level.

Movement

- As you exhale, press rope down-ward until your arms are straight, but unlocked.

- While pressing down, move your hands apart so that, at the end of the ROM, your hands will be adjacent to your thighs.
- Hold contraction for $1/2$ second.
- Slowly raise your forearms while inhaling, bringing your hands chest-level.

Helpful hints

- Maintain firm abs.
- Always keep your neck and shoulders relaxed.
- Avoid leaning forward as you press down.
- Keep your wrists straight.

French Press (Nose Crunchers)

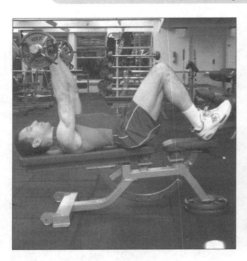 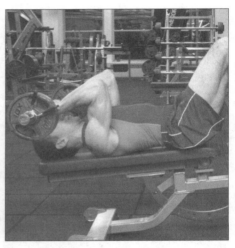

Muscles worked

- *Primary:* Triceps (all three heads).
- *Support:* Front delts and abs.

Positioning

- Place bench at a slight decline angle—twenty to twenty-five degrees. You can use a couple of weight plates to raise one end of the bench.
- Holding an E-Z barbell, sit on the elevated edge of bench, placing barbell on thighs.
- As you lie back onto the bench, use your legs to propel the barbell into position over your chest.
- Hold arms straight up towards ceiling, with elbows pointed toward knees.
- Place the heels of your feet on the bench.

Movement

- As you exhale, press the barbell upward until your arms are straight, but unlocked (keep elbows pointed toward your knees throughout the ROM).
- Hold in the top position momentarily.
- Slowly lower the barbell while inhaling, bringing the barbell just above your nose.

Helpful hints

- Maintain a bend at your knees.
- Keep your elbows pointed up toward the ceiling (avoid rocking your upper arms forward and backward).
- Keep your wrists straight at all times.

Cable Kickback

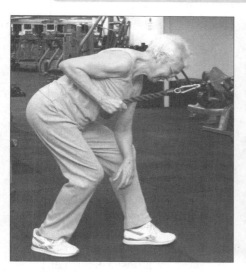
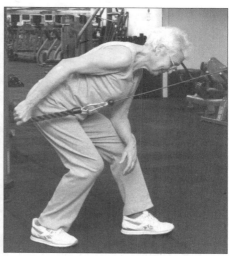

Muscles worked

- *Primary:* Outer triceps.
- *Support:* Center triceps, rear delts, and abs.

Positioning

- Place cable pulley to setting at waistline height.
- Holding a rope grip, step two feet back from machine.
- Stand with feet hip-width apart.
- Move foot of working side back by two to three feet, getting into a semi-lunge position.
- Lean forward, resting non-working arm on leg of the same side.
- Raise elbow of working arm to a horizontal position, adjacent to torso.
- Position elbow of working arm at a sixty- to seventy-degree angle.

Movement

- As you exhale, press rope backward until your arm is straight, but unlocked (keep elbow to your side).
- Hold in the extended position momentarily.
- Slowly lower your forearm while inhaling, returning your hand to the beginning position.

Helpful hints

- Keep the upper portion of your working arm in one position, parallel to the floor (avoid rocking it up and down).
- Keep your head and neck in a straight line with your upper back (avoid looking up).
- Keep your wrist straight at all times.

Dumbbell Kickbacks

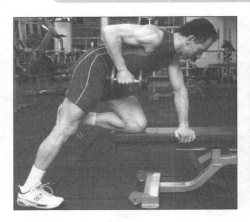 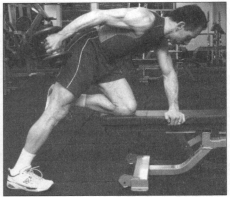

Muscles worked

- *Primary:* Outer triceps.

- *Support:* Center triceps, rear delts, and abs.

Positioning

- Position the knee and hand of your non-working side onto a bench (to protect your wrist, turn your hand inward so your fingers hang over the edge of the bench toward your midline).

- Place the foot of your working side on the floor behind you, and close to your opposite leg.

- Keep your back flat (horizontal) and your shoulders and hips, parallel.

- Holding a weight in your working hand, raise elbow and upper arm to a horizontal position adjacent to torso.

- Maintain an angle of sixty- to seventy-degrees at the elbow.

Movement

- As you exhale, press weight upward until your arm is straight, but unlocked (keep elbow to your side).

- Hold in the elevated position momentarily.

- Slowly lower the weight while inhaling, bringing your hand to the beginning position.

Helpful hints

- Maintain firm abs.

- Keep the upper portion of your working arm in one position, parallel to the floor (avoid rocking it up and down).

- Keep your head and neck in a straight line with your upper back (avoid looking up).

- Avoid locking out your elbows and your knee on the working side.

- Keep your wrist straight at all times.

13

Exercises—
Core Body

The core region of the body is where all strength and balance originates. For optimal functioning in everyday tasks, including physical activities, and the prevention of injuries—as well as improved aesthetics—it is critical that the core region be conditioned. The core consists primarily of two interrelated areas: the abdominals and the lower back (erector) muscles. For this region of the body, I do not encourage the use of machines. Instead, I recommend sticking with the calisthenic exercises described in this chapter.

Abdominals

For the abdominals, there are four layers of muscles. In order of outermost (external) to innermost layers, they are: *rectus abdominus, external obliques, internal obliques,* and *transverse abdominus.*

Rectus Abdominus

The rectus abdominus is a band of muscles running vertically along your central torso, attached (at the top end) to the bottom or your rib cage and (at the bottom end) to the top of your pelvic bone. This muscle group is where the six-pack muscles (whether or not you can see them) are situated. While this muscle group is primarily responsible for spinal flexion (bending forward), it also allows for spinal extension (bending backward) and assists the obliques with torso rotation—from a rotated position back to neutral.

External and Internal Obliques

The obliques (also known as love handles) are muscles positioned on the sides of the torso, angled at forty-five-degrees from the rectus abdominis. External obliques are angled downward, at the same angle as if you were to put your hands in your pants pockets. Internal obliques are angled upward. Both layers work synergistically to twist the torso in either direction and to assist the main abs region in flexing the torso.

Transverse Abdominus

The transverse abdominis, the innermost layer of the abdominals, is positioned horizontally, wrapping around the torso and attaching to the spine. This muscle group is most directly related to spinal and torso stabilization, as well as biological functioning (elimination, breathing).

Upper, Obliques, and Lower Abdominal Exercises

Although my preference is to divide abdominal exercises into three groups—upper, obliques, and lower—take note that, anatomically (structurally), there is actually no separation of upper and lower abs. What is commonly referred to as upper and lower abs is all one band of muscle tissue—rectus abdominis. However, physiologically (functionally), the upper and lower portions of this one band of muscle have both overlapping and separate functions. Depending

ATTAINING SIX-PACK ABS

Whether or not you can see your six-pack muscles, they are there. Two variables are involved: How much body fat you have and how conditioned your abs are. The exercises in this chapter will help you tone and condition your abdominal muscles. They won't, however, help to burn any fat. One of the main myths discussed in Chapter 1 is that there's no such thing as spot-reducing fat. So eat right (avoid saturated fats and simple sugars), do cardio exercises (they burn the most calories per minute of exercise), lift weights (this helps increase muscle tissue, which directly eats fat), and do your abdominal exercises (shape and tone your mid-section).

on the movement involved, some exercises place more emphasis on the lower abs, while other movements place more emphasis on the upper abs.

More specifically, when the lower body moves (as in a knee-up movement), lower abs are primarily affected. When the upper body moves (as in a crunch upward, or forward, if standing), upper abs are the focus.

The philosophy of working larger muscles first and smaller muscles last applies to abdominal exercising. Always work your lower abs first, obliques second, and upper abs last. When challenging the lower abs, you are also recruiting support from your upper abs. But when you work your upper abs, you are focusing almost exclusively on that area. Therefore, if you begin your abs routine by working your upper abs first (the most common mistake in abs conditioning), then you will pre-fatigue that area, thereby diminishing your ability to properly challenge lower abs.

As you will notice, there are no exercises involving a full sitting up movement. This is because a situp, or any exercise that involves full ninety-degree flexion of the hips, pulls on the lower back via hip-flexor muscles. Hip flexors are attached to the lower vertebrae and will stress them more than the abs will be challenged. While it is good to challenge the hip flexors, this is not the ideal way to do that.

The eight ab exercises taught in this book are more than enough for you to begin a routine that will help strengthen and flatten your abs. If you have already been challenging your ab region, you can add a couple of exercises that are new for you to your routine.

Back Extensors

The official names for back extensors are *erector spinae* and *multifidus*. These are the primary muscle movers for back extension (bending backward) and rotation. They also are primarily responsible for keeping the torso upright, preventing it from buckling forward.

These muscles, in concert with the abdominals, are responsible for helping you to function optimally and prevent pain and injury. Here are some general exercise suggestions.

• Avoid fast, jerking movements.

• Always keep your neck and shoulders as relaxed and uninvolved as possible.

- Avoid pulling on your head with your hands. Use your hands simply to carry the weight of your head. When done properly, your hands can help keep your neck as relaxed as when your head is resting on a pillow.

- On the downward, or return, movement of each exercise, continue using your abs to lower your body (this protects your lower back from overarching and being overstressed). Keep the back of your rib cage pressed to the floor, while maintaining a slight arc at your lower back.

- Always exhale on the upward movement. This allows for more efficient breathing, as well as stronger ab contractions.

CHOOSING THE RIGHT STABILITY BALL SIZE

Select a stability ball size where you can maintain a 90-degree angle at your knees while sitting on the ball. Use the table below to determine the best size ball based on your height.

Your Height	Ball Diameter
Up to 5'4"	45 cm.
5'5" to 5'7"	55 cm.
5'8" to 6'0"	65 cm.
Over 6'0"	75 cm.

ABDOMINALS

LOWER ABS

Reverse Crunch 🏠

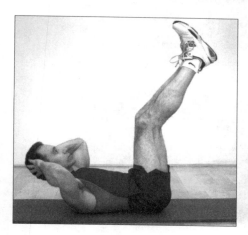
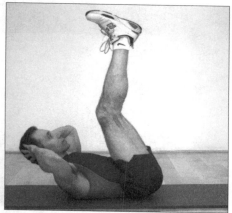

Muscles worked

- *Primary:* Lower and mid abs.

- *Support:* Upper abs.

Positioning

- Lie down on your back, in a supine (face-up) position.

- Position both hands under your head.

- Raise head and shoulders up, off the floor.

- Raise legs up, pointing feet toward the ceiling, positioning your knees directly over hips.

Movement

- As you exhale, contract your lower and mid abs, pulling your legs toward your chin.

- Move your legs through a thirty-degree ROM.

- While inhaling, use your lower and mid abs to return your legs to the beginning position.

Helpful hints

- Avoid using momentum to move your legs.

- Initiate the movement from your lower and mid abs—avoid using leg muscles to move your legs.

Toe Taps 🏠

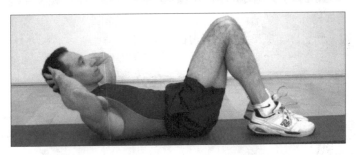

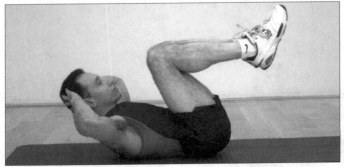

Muscles worked

- *Primary:* Lower and mid abs.
- *Support:* Upper abs.

Positioning

- Lie down on your back, face-up.
- Position both hands under your head.
- Raise head and shoulders up, off the floor.
- Maintain bend at knees.
- Keep heels about six to eight inches away from butt.

Movement

- As you exhale, contract your lower and mid abs, pulling your knees toward your chest.
- Move your legs through a thirty to forty-degree ROM, stopping when your knees are over your chest.
- While inhaling, use your lower and mid abs to return your legs to the beginning position.

Helpful hints

- Keep neck and shoulders relaxed.
- Initiate the movement from your lower and mid abs—avoid using leg muscles to move your legs.

OBLIQUES

One-Sided Obliques

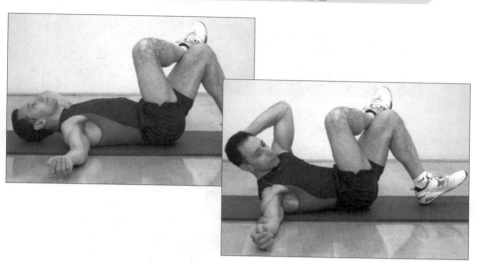

Muscles worked

• *Primary:* Obliques and upper abs.

Positioning

• Lie down on your back, face-up.

• Keep your right knee bent.

• Position your left ankle across your right knee.

• Rest your head on your right palm.

• Extend your left arm onto the floor, out to your left.

Movement

• As you exhale, contract your abs and obliques—particularly along your left side—to raise your right shoulder toward your left knee.

• Move your torso upward and over by thirty degrees.

• While inhaling, slowly, lower your torso to the beginning position.

• After performing a complete set of repetitions, switch sides.

Helpful hints

• Keep the weight of your head rested in your palm.

• Keep your elbow pointed out to the side as you move through the ROM—twist from your torso (using obliques) without flapping your elbow forward.

• For greater intensity, slightly raise the hip you're turning toward, bringing your opposite hip and shoulder slightly toward each other.

Alternate Oblique Twists 🏠

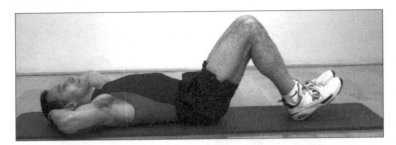

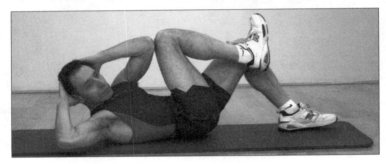

Muscles worked

- *Primary:* Obliques and upper abs.

Positioning

- Lie down on your back, face-up.
- Keep both knees bent.
- Rest your head on your palms.
- For added back support, keep your toes pointed up, with your heels resting on the floor.

Movement

- While exhaling, contract your abs and obliques as you raise your left elbow and right knee toward each other.
- Contract your upper torso upward and over to the right by thirty degrees or until your elbow and knee touch; simultaneously contract your lower torso over toward the left.
- While inhaling, slowly lower your torso to the beginning position.
- As you exhale, contract your abs and work the alternate obliques, moving your right elbow and left knee toward each other.

Helpful hints

- With each rep, return your torso to the original position before performing your next rep.
- For a maximal contraction, as you advance, have your moving elbow tap the outside of your opposite knee.

Ball Obliques (Advanced) 🏠

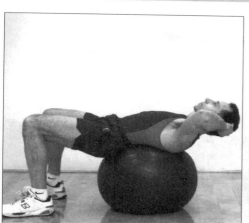
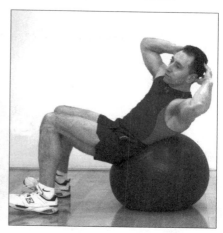

Muscles worked

• *Primary:* Obliques, upper abs, transverse abdominus, and stabilizers.

Positioning

• Choose appropriate stability ball size. (See sidebar on page 158.)

• Sit upright on the ball.

• Step by step, walk forward, lowering your back onto the ball.

• Move forward until your mid back is on the ball.

• Keep your torso straight (avoid overarching).

• Position your feet at shoulder-width distance.

Movement

• While exhaling, contract your abs and squeeze your left obliques as you raise your torso and twist toward your left hip.

• Contract and twist your torso until your right shoulder is facing toward your left hip.

• While inhaling, slowly lower your torso to the beginning position.

• While exhaling, contract your abs and the alternate obliques as you turn in the alternate direction.

Helpful hints

• If this exercise is too challenging, then ease the intensity by positioning the ball under your upper back.

• For beginners, keep your feet wider than shoulder-width distance (easier balance).

• For advanced, keep your feet closer than shoulder width for less stability.

UPPER ABS

Crunch—Straight Arms

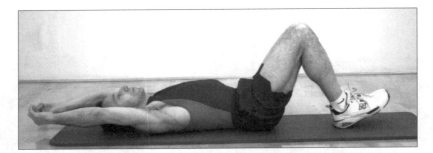

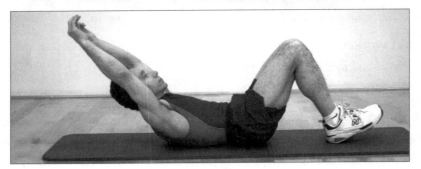

Muscles worked

- *Primary:* Upper abs.

Positioning

- Lie down on your back, face-up.
- Keep both knees bent and toes pointed up (for added back support).
- Keep your arms straight and adjacent to your head.

Movement

- As you exhale, crunch upward, keeping your arms adjacent to your head.
- Move your torso upward by thirty degrees.
- While inhaling, slowly lower your torso to the beginning position.

Helpful hints

- If your neck begins to fatigue, or if you generally have tight neck muscles, keep one hand under your head to carry the weight of your head.
- Keep your rear rib cage pressed to the floor.

Crunch (Basic) 🏠

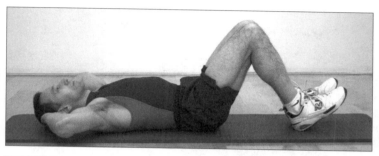

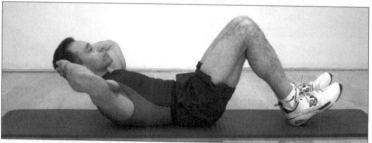

Muscles worked

• *Primary:* Upper abs.

Positioning

• Lie down on your back, face-up.

• Keep both knees bent.

• Rest your head on your palms.

• For added back support, keep your toes pointed up, with your heels resting on the floor.

Movement

• As you exhale, contract your abs, moving your torso upward.

• Move upward by thirty degrees.

• Hold torso in the up position momentarily.

• As you inhale, slowly lower your torso to the beginning position while keeping your lower rib cage pressed to the floor.

Helpful hints

• Keep the weight of your head rested in your palms.

• Keep your elbows pointed out to the sides as you move through the ROM, without flapping your elbows forward.

• Keep your chin away from your chest—imagine having a tennis ball under your chin.

Ball Crunch (Advanced) 🏠

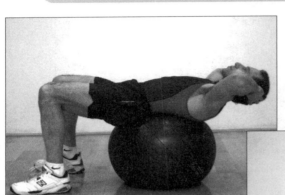

Muscles worked

- *Primary:* Upper abs and stabilizers.

Positioning

- Choose appropriate stability ball size. (See sidebar on page 158.)
- Sit upright on the ball.
- Step by step, walk forward, lowering your back onto the ball.
- Move forward until your mid back is on the ball.
- Keep your torso straight.
- Position your feet at shoulder-width distance.

Movement

- While exhaling, contract your abs as you raise your torso upward.
- Move your torso upward by thirty degrees, keeping your hips level (prevent them from pressing down).
- While inhaling, slowly lower your torso to the beginning position.

Helpful hints

- If this exercise is too challenging, then begin by positioning the ball under your upper back.
- For beginners, keep your feet wider than shoulder-width distance (better balance).
- For advanced, keep your feet closer than shoulder width.

BACK EXTENSORS

Bridge Extension

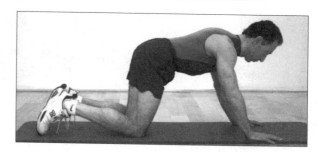

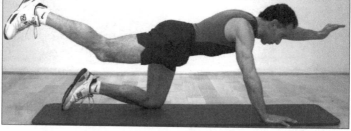

Muscles worked

• *Primary:* Erector spinae and multifidus—muscles that run along both sides of the spine.

• *Support:* Abs, triceps, deltoids, glutes, and hamstrings.

Positioning

• Get into the all-four's (bridge) position—rest on your hands and knees.

• Position your wrists under your shoulders.

• Position your knees under your hips.

• Keep your head in a straight line with your torso.

• Keep your back straight.

Movement

• As you exhale, extend only your left arm forward into a straightened position and hold for two seconds.

• Inhale as you lower your arm to the beginning position.

• Extend your right leg straight back and hold for two seconds.

• Lower to the beginning position.

• Extend your right arm and hold for two seconds.

• Extend your left leg and hold for two seconds.

Helpful hints

• When this exercise becomes easy, simultaneously raise opposite limbs (alternate left arm and right leg, then right arm and left leg).

• Prevent your lower back from sagging downward.

• Prevent your chin from dropping down toward your chest or the floor.

Prone Limb Raises 🏠

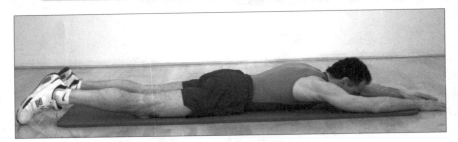

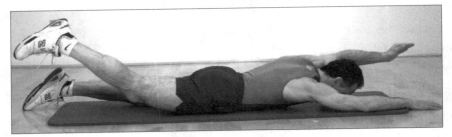

Muscles worked

- *Primary:* Erector spinae and multifidus.
- *Support:* Abs, deltoids, glutes, and hamstrings.

Positioning

- Lie down in a prone (face-down) position.
- Extend arms out, overhead and on the floor.

Movement

- As you exhale, raise only your left arm upward, in a straightened position, as high as you comfortably can.
- Hold for two seconds.
- Inhale as you lower your arm to the beginning position.

- Raise your right leg (starting from your hip) straight up, as far as you comfortably can.
- Hold for two seconds.
- Lower to the beginning position.
- Raise your right arm and hold for two seconds.
- Raise your left leg and hold for two seconds.

Helpful hints

- When this exercise becomes easy, simultaneously raise opposite limbs (alternate right arm and left leg, then left arm and right leg).
- Prevent your lower back from overarching.
- Avoid pressing your chin into the floor.

Hyperextensions

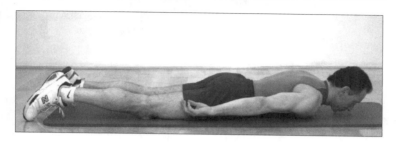

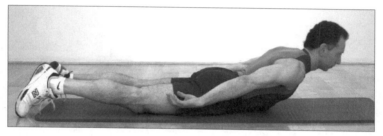

Muscles worked

- *Primary:* Erector spinae and multifidus.
- *Support:* Abs, glutes, and hamstrings.

Positioning

- Lie down in a prone (face-down) position.
- Keep your arms by the sides of your body.

Movement

- As you exhale, raise your torso upward by one to two inches and hold for two seconds.
- Inhale as you lower your torso to the beginning position.
- Raise your right leg straight up and hold for two seconds.
- Lower to the beginning position.
- Raise your left leg and hold for two seconds.

Helpful hints

- When this exercise becomes easy, alternately raise your right leg, then your left leg with each rep that you raise your torso.
- For an even greater challenge, raise both legs as you raise your torso.
- Keep your neck and shoulders relaxed.

14

Exercises— Flexibility

In order to live a fully functioning lifestyle, it is critical to attain and maintain a good level of flexibility. Loss of flexibility (and strength) greatly affects balance, coordination, and movement. While many feel that a loss of flexibility is simply a symptom of advancing age, rest assured that these losses are more related to inactivity than chronological aging.

The Need for Flexibility

In many ways, it's the classic Catch 22. People are told they can do less as they get older, so they actually *do* less. Meanwhile, doing less leads to inactivity, and inactivity leads to loss of flexibility, which leads to, you guessed it, doing even less—the proverbial vicious cycle. Regardless of age, *active* people tend to be more flexible and better balanced than their *inactive* counterparts.

Flexibility conditioning, otherwise known as stretching, has been specifically designed here to enhance the performance of day-to-day tasks. As such, it should be an integral part of any health and fitness program. Even for weight training, flexibility is needed to increase your strength level. When a muscle or muscle group is tight, its strength potential becomes limited.

An important concept to understand when considering flexibility exercises is range of motion (ROM). This is the ability to *safely* go through the full range of possible movement around a joint. I stress the word safely because many people, stuck on the dangerous notion that more is better, tend to force their bodies beyond their true ROM and, in the process, wind up doing more harm than good . . . to themselves, that is.

Several times a week, I notice people at the gym who push their stretches beyond a particular joint's capacity. In effect, they *force* their bodies into various contorted stretches and positions—ones the human body wasn't necessarily designed to handle.

Too Much of a Good Thing

The purpose of this chapter is not just to present details as to what types of stretching are ideal and how to do them, but also to advise you of the potential problems associated with stretching—in terms of stretching too far, too much, or even at the wrong times of day or night. Contrary to what you may have been taught, I must warn you that too much stretching, and even stretching *before* an activity, will not help prevent injury. In fact, both may actually increase your chances for injury.

A recent review of the latest stretching research, as reported in the *Physician and Sports Medicine* magazine, indicated that the "results of many of the studies on stretching are contradictory, inconclusive, or not necessarily applicable to humans." In fact, it goes on to suggest that "stretching immediately before exercise does not prevent overuse or acute injuries."

When it comes to stretching, as related to health and fitness, even too much of a *good* thing can be quite *bad*. As important as it is, stretching has been overrated in the past.

I know what your old football coach, gym owner, or best friend, Sally, the fast-walker, told you, but there is a time and a place for everything. Far from helping the situation, overstretching may actually contribute to a loss in joint stability. Stretching before starting an activity has been shown to be negligible when it comes to preventing injuries, and new studies show it may actually increase the potential for injury.

In addition to that fabled flexibility-producer of old, stretching, there is another great method to increase flexibility: Yoga. However, even with Yoga, there are a few sticking points. Several exercises force the body into unnatural postures which, in turn, force the body to go beyond its normal ROM.

Two specific examples are: The *cobra*—the posture where the body is arched backwards while the hips and legs rest on the floor; and the *plough,* whereby the body is in a supine (face-up position), and the legs are raised up and over, bringing the toes overhead to touch the floor. The first exercise places a tremendous amount of stress on the lumbar (lower back) spine, while the latter stresses the cervical (neck) vertebrae by placing too much of the body's weight on such a small—not to mention sensitive—area. Any yogini knows it takes a great deal of practice under the supervision of a skilled practitioner to successfully work into these postures, and beginners need to be aware of that.

Ignore the fads and old wives' tales and remember this: Good stretching occurs by knowing your own body. Not your neighbors' bodies, not mine, and not the buffed instructor on your stack of exercise videos.

Stretching has nothing to do with how far you can move a specific joint or how far your toes can go beyond your nose. In my opinion, being able to touch your head to your heels behind you, for example, serves no purpose in everyday life. Stretching routines should be individualized and personalized according to the individual's physical structure and conditioning level.

Exercise Techniques

The seventeen variations of exercises covered in this chapter are broken down into two segments: pre- and post-workout stretches, and intra-workout stretches. The pre-workout stretches should not be considered warmups, but should instead be performed after a warmup. An ideal warmup would consist of an aerobic exercise performed briskly for six to ten minutes.

While the primary purpose of pre- and post-workout stretches is to limber up, all the stretches presented in this chapter are designed to help you achieve more flexibility and better balance in a safe, effective manner. Such exercises help make basic functioning more natural and efficient. Here are some suggestions for developing more flexibility.

- Breathe through each exercise—avoid breath-holding. Inhale while your muscles are relaxed. Exhale as you ease into, and maintain, your maximal stretch.

- Avoid locking out joints. Bring each stretch through a full ROM, stopping just prior to hyperextending the joint.

- Hold each stretch for two to three long counts. For example, count a two-second stretch as follows: one Mississippi, two Mississippi.

- Perform between three and eight repetitions of each stretch.

- Avoid bouncing (ballistic) movements.

And now, here are those flexibility exercises, divided into pre- and post-workout stretches and intra-workout (during the workout) stretches.

PRE- AND POST-WORKOUT STRETCHES

Supine Press

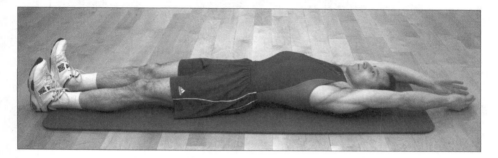

Muscles stretched

- Back and abs.

Positioning

- Lie down in a supine (face-up) position.
- Keep knees straight, and legs rested on floor.
- Straighten out elbows and keep arms adjacent to your head.

Movement

- As you exhale, press your legs and arms in opposite directions, along the horizontal plane (legs press downward and arms press overhead).
- Hold stretch for two to three long counts.
- While inhaling, ease out of stretch.
- Perform three to five reps.

Helpful hints

- Keep neck and shoulders relaxed, even as your press your limbs in opposite directions.
- Avoid pressing your head and/or heels down into the floor.

Supine Press with Arc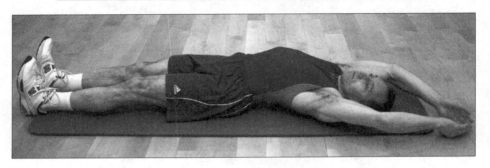

Muscles stretched

- Back and abs.

Positioning

- Lie down in a supine (face-up) position.
- Keep knees straight, and legs rested on floor.
- Straighten out elbows and keep arms adjacent to your head.

Movement

- As you exhale, press your right leg and right arm in opposite directions along the horizontal plane (leg presses downward and arm presses overhead).
- Slightly reach over toward the left with your right hand as you press your arm and leg on the right side; arc your body toward the left side.
- Hold stretch for two long counts.
- While inhaling, ease out of stretch.
- Stretch/arc toward the opposite direction.
- Perform three to five reps on alternate sides.

Helpful hints

- Keep neck and shoulders relaxed, even as you press your limbs in opposite directions.
- Avoid pressing your head and/or heels down into the floor.

Knee Hugs 🏠

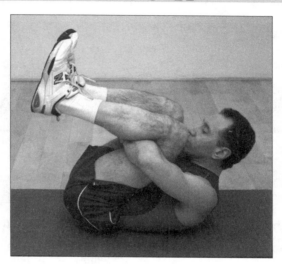

Muscles stretched

- Back.

Positioning

- Lie down in a supine (face-up) position.
- Hug your knees to your chest.
- Hold your legs from under the knees (this prevents any unnecessary stress on the knees).
- Bring your chin to your knees.

Movement

- As you exhale, pull your legs and chest in toward each other.
- Hold stretch for two long counts.
- While inhaling, ease out of stretch, bringing your feet and back to the floor.
- Perform three to five reps.

Helpful hints

- Be sure to continue breathing as you hold your stretch.
- For additional stretching, add a slight side-to-side rocking motion as you hold each stretch.
- When lowering your feet and head to the floor, keep the rear of your rib cage pressed to the floor.

Knees-to-Side 🏠

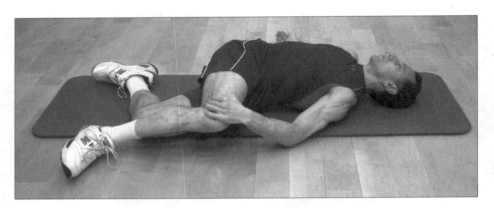

Muscles stretched

- Lats, lower back, and/or hips.

Positioning

- Lie down in a supine (face-up) position.
- Keep feet on the mat with knees bent.
- Bring arms out to the sides.

Movement

- As you exhale, lower your knees to the left.

- Extend your right (upper) leg slightly beyond the lower (left) leg—this allows for a deeper stretch.
- Place your left hand above your right knee and press gently.
- Hold stretch for two long counts.
- While inhaling, ease out of stretch, bringing your knees to the center.
- Switch sides to do the inverse.
- Perform three to five reps, alternating sides.

Helpful hints

- If this stretch is too strong, then keep your knees together throughout the stretch.
- If you are very limber, straighten your lower leg and maintain only a slight bend at the upper knee.

Cat-Backs/Camel-Backs 🏠

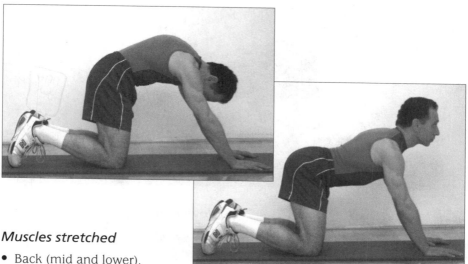

Muscles stretched

• Back (mid and lower).

Positioning

• Get into a *bridge* position—rest on your hands and knees.

• Position your wrists under your shoulders.

• Position your knees under your hips.

• Keep your head in a straight line with your torso.

• Keep your back straight.

Movement

• While exhaling, pull your abs in as you curl your back upward.

• Lower your head downward.

• Hold stretch for two long counts.

• While inhaling, ease out of stretch, lowering your abs toward the floor.

• Gently arc your back downward as you raise your chin to look up.

• Perform three to five reps.

Helpful hints

• In the cat-back position (back curled upward), avoid tightening your neck and shoulder muscles.

• In the camel-back position, avoid pressing your abs toward the floor.

Kneeling Bow

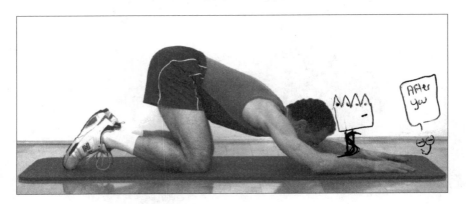

Muscles stretched

• Upper back (postural muscles) and rear delts.

Positioning

• Get into a *bridge* position—rest on your hands and knees.

• Walk your hands forward so they are eight to twelve inches ahead of your shoulders.

Movement

• As you exhale, shift your hips back toward your heels.

• Raise your chin upward.

• Gently press your chest downward.

• Hold stretch for two long counts.

• While inhaling, ease out of stretch, moving back to the bridge position.

• Perform three to five reps.

Helpful hints

• Avoid pressing down too heavily.

• If you have shoulder sensitivities or rotator cuff injuries, avoid this exercise.

INTRA-WORKOUT STRETCHES

UPPER BODY

Chest (With Thumb Up) 🏠

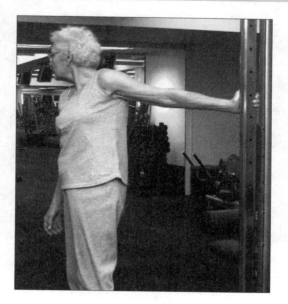

Positioning

- Place your left hand against a pole or wall, thumb-up.
- Keep hand at chest level.
- Position feet hip-width apart.
- Maintain slight bend at knees.

Movement

- As you exhale, slowly turn torso toward right.
- Hold stretch for two long counts.
- While inhaling, ease out of stretch.
- Perform three to five reps prior to switching sides.

Helpful hints

- Keep elbows and knees unlocked.
- In between reps, let go of pole and contract pecs—perform imaginary chest press.

Back (Main—Both Lats)

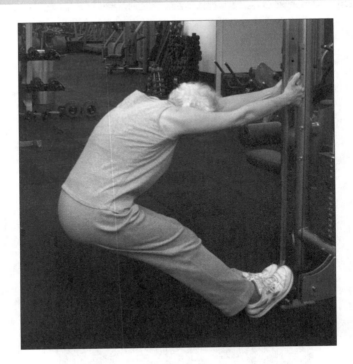

Positioning

• Place both feet against bottom of pole.

• Clasp pole with both hands at waist level.

Movement

• While exhaling, slowly bring hips backward, straightening out arms and legs.

• Dip head between arms.

• Stop just prior to locking out elbows and knees.

• Allow your body weight to shift towards your buttocks.

Helpful hints

• To fully stretch, keep your neck, shoulders, arms, and back as relaxed as possible.

Back (Single Lat)

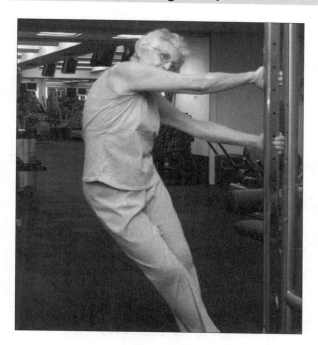

Positioning

• Standing adjacent to a pole or archway, with your left side closer to it, place your right hand high on the pole (slightly above shoulder height).

• Position your left hand several inches below your right hand.

• Place your right foot against the bottom of the pole.

• Place your left foot behind your right foot.

Movement

• As you exhale, slowly arc your body away from the pole, tilting your hips outward, bringing your body into a C-shaped posture.

• Move your right hip outward until you feel a strong stretch along your right lat muscles.

• Hold stretch for two long counts.

• While inhaling, ease out of stretch as you return to the original upright position.

• Perform three to five reps prior to switching sides.

Helpful hints

• Keep elbows and knees unlocked.

• In between reps, contract your lats, squeezing your shoulder blades toward each other.

Shoulders (Deltoids) 🏠

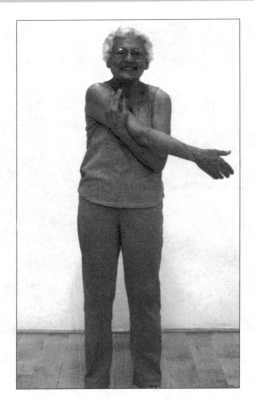

Positioning

- Stand with feet hip-width apart.
- Bring right arm across your chest, while keeping your shoulder and neck muscles relaxed.
- Position left wrist just above right elbow, with your left palm facing you.

Movement

- As you exhale, slowly pull on your right arm with your left wrist.
- Hold stretch for two long counts.
- While inhaling, release your right arm.
- Perform three to five reps prior to switching sides.

Helpful hints

- Always keep your stretching arm limber.
- In between reps, release arm and perform an imaginary shoulder press.

Biceps (with Thumb Down) 🏠

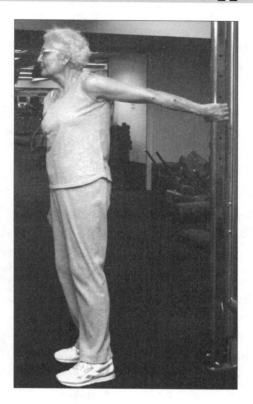

Positioning

- Clasp a pole (or side of a door) with your left hand, thumb down.
- Keep hand at chest level.
- Position feet hip-width apart.

Movement

- As you exhale, slowly turn torso toward right side.
- Hold stretch for two long counts.
- While inhaling, ease out of stretch.
- Perform three to five reps prior to switching sides.

Helpful hints

- Keep elbows and knees unlocked.
- In between reps, let go of pole and contract biceps—perform imaginary bicep curl.

Triceps 🏠

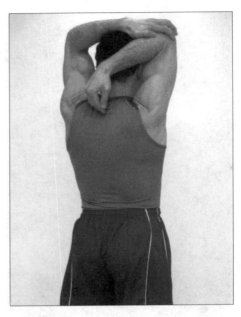

Positioning

• Stand with feet hip-width apart.

• Bring right arm overhead, with hand behind neck (like scratching your upper back).

• Place left hand on right elbow.

Movement

• As you exhale, slowly pull on your right elbow with your left hand.

• Hold stretch for two long counts.

• While inhaling, release your right arm.

• Perform three to five reps prior to switching sides.

Helpful hints

• For a deeper stretch, contract your biceps as you stretch the triceps.

• In between reps, release arm and perform an imaginary triceps extension (straighten arm).

LOWER BODY

Hamstrings (Rear Thighs) 🏠

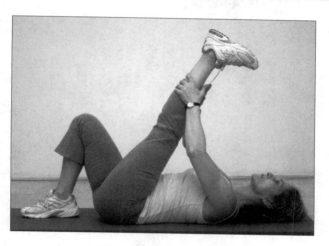

Positioning

• Lie down on your back, facing up.

• Bend your right knee, keeping your left leg straight and resting on the floor.

Movement

• As you exhale, raise your left leg upward.

• Slightly flex your foot downward so your toes point down toward your nose.

• Keeping your leg straight, hold your leg either above or below the knee.

• Pull gently until you feel a strong stretch behind your knee and/or along the back of your thigh.

• Hold stretch for two long counts.

• While inhaling, release your left leg, slowly lowering it to the floor.

• Perform three to five reps prior to switching sides.

Helpful hints

• For a deeper stretch, contract your quads as you stretch the hamstrings.

• Avoid bending the knee of your stretching leg.

Quadriceps (Front Thighs) 🏠

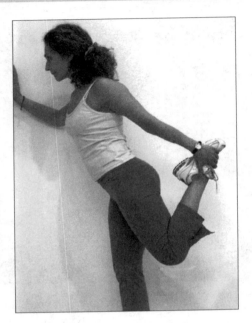

Positioning

- Stand two to three feet away from a wall or exercise machine.
- Hold onto it with your right hand.

Movement

- As you exhale, raise your left foot back toward your buttocks.
- Hold your left ankle with your left hand.
- Lean forward as you pull your leg back further, pressing your heel upward.
- Pull gently until you feel a strong stretch on the front of your thigh.

- Hold stretch for two long counts.
- While inhaling, release your left leg, returning it to the starting position.
- Perform three to five reps prior to switching sides.

Helpful hints

- For a deeper stretch, contract your hamstrings and glutes as you stretch the quads.
- Avoid hyperflexing the knee (pressing heel to butt) of your stretching leg.

Abductors 🏠

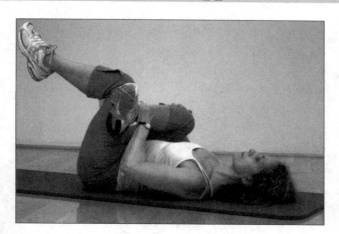

Positioning

- Lie down on your back.

- Bend your left knee, keeping your left foot on the floor.

- Bring your right ankle across your left thigh (just above the knee).

Movement

- As you exhale, raise your left leg upward.

- Hold your right leg both at the ankle and the knee.

- Pull your right leg toward your chest until you feel a strong stretch along the outer thigh and butt region of your right leg.

- Hold stretch for two long counts.

- While inhaling, release both legs, slowly lowering your left foot to the floor.

- Perform three to five reps prior to switching sides.

Helpful hints

- For a deeper stretch, use both hands as well as your resting leg to pull your stretching leg into position.

- In between reps, extend your stretching leg into a straightened position while contracting your glutes.

Adductors 🏠

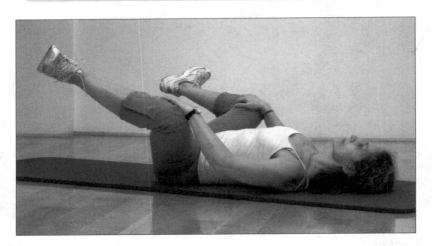

Positioning

• Lie down on your back.

• Keeping knees bent, bring them both over your hips.

• Place your hands on the insides of your thighs (just above the knees).

Movement

• As you exhale, lower your legs outward to the sides.

• Stop moving out and downward when you feel a strong stretch at your inner thigh and groin muscles.

• Slightly and gently, press both legs downward with your hands.

• Hold stretch for two long counts.

• While inhaling, bring your legs back together, positioning them above your hips.

• Perform three to five reps.

Helpful hints

• For a deeper stretch, contract your glutes as you press your legs downward.

• If your inner thigh and groin muscles are tight, simply place your hands on your legs without pressing down—the weight of your hands will provide a sufficient stretch.

Calves 🏠

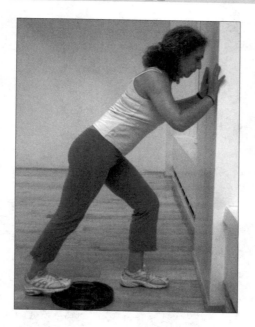

Positioning

- Stand in front of a stationary object (e.g., a wall or park bench).
- Place your left foot in front of you.
- Place your right foot behind you, keeping the ball and toes of that foot on a slightly elevated object (one to two inches high).

Movement

- As you exhale, lean forward, shifting your body weight onto your left leg.
- While doing this, press your right heel into the floor.
- Keep your right knee in a semi-locked position.
- Hold stretch for two long counts.
- While inhaling, relax your right leg.
- Perform three to five reps prior to switching sides.

Helpful hints

- In between reps, contract your stretching calf, raising heel off the floor.

Achilles Tendon

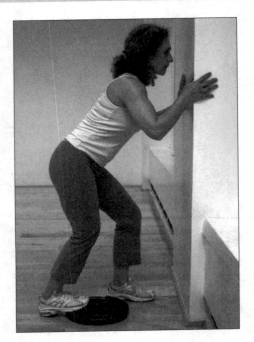

Positioning

- Stand in front of a stationary object (e.g., a wall or park bench).
- Place your left foot slightly in front of your right foot.
- Keep the ball and toes of right foot on a slightly elevated object (one to two inches high).
- Bring right leg into a semi-squat position.

Movement

- As you exhale, lean forward while shifting your body weight onto your right heel.
- While doing this, press your right heel into the floor.
- Hold stretch for two long counts.
- While inhaling, relax your right leg.
- Perform three to five reps prior to switching sides.

Helpful hints

- In between reps, contract your stretching calf, raising heel off the floor.

Anterior Tibialis (Front Shin) 🏠

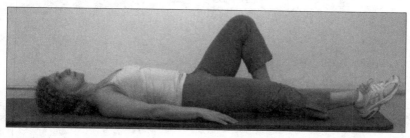

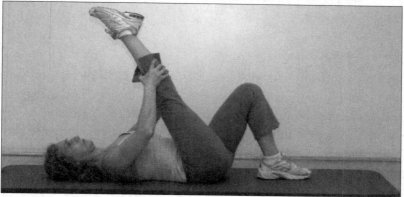

Positioning

• Lie down on your back, facing up.

• Bend your left knee, while keeping your right leg straight and resting on the floor.

Movement

• As you exhale, raise your right leg upward.

• Point your toes toward ceiling.

• Keeping your leg straight, hold your leg from either above or below the knee.

• Pull gently until you feel a strong stretch on your right instep (front of ankle).

• Hold stretch for two long counts.

• While inhaling, release your right leg, slowly lowering it to the floor.

• Perform three to five reps prior to switching legs.

Helpful hints

• For a deeper stretch, contract your calf muscles as you stretch the shin muscles.

• Avoid bending the knee of your stretching leg.

15

Exercises—
Balance

Although improvements in strength and flexibility indirectly enhance balance, it is important to perform exercises that specifically challenge balance capabilities. As people age, moving into their sixties, seventies, or eighties, bone fractures become more of a threat to well-being than any other ailment.

Broken bones result from falls that are more of a common occurrence due to losses in balance capabilities. Balance, therefore, becomes more and more of a priority in maintaining a higher quality of life. The exercises in this chapter (seven variations) will help you to maintain or improve your equilibrium and thus maintain independent living all through life. Even if you are nowhere near your sixties, balance training will still benefit you in your daily activities.

Toes To Heels (Part 1)

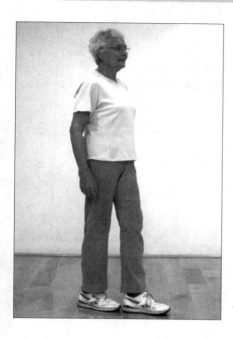

- Stand upright, with shoulders over hips, hips over knees, and knees over ankles.

- Position left foot in front of right foot so the toes of your right foot are touching the heel of your left.

- Keep both knees straight. Have your weight evenly distributed on both legs.

- Initially, you may need to hold on to a sturdy object for balance. However, as you improve your balance with this exercise, keep both hands at your sides.

- After several seconds, switch sides.

- When this exercise becomes easier, or when you can hold this basic position for thirty seconds or more, challenge yourself further by doing the next variation.

Toes To Heels (Part 2)

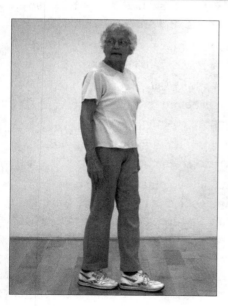

- Position left foot in front of right foot so the toes of your right foot are touching the heel of your left.

- Look over one shoulder for two to three seconds. Then look over the other shoulder for two to three seconds.

- Perform three to five alternating repetitions before switching sides.

- When this becomes easier, you may proceed to the next variation.

Toes To Heels (Part 3) 🏠

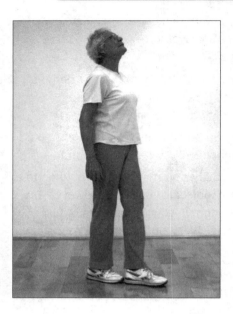

- Position left foot in front of right foot so the toes of your right foot are touching the heel of your left.

- Look straight up, overhead, for two to three seconds.

- Perform three to five repetitions.

- When this becomes easier, perform the first variation (Part 1) with your eyes closed.

Standing Abduction 🏠

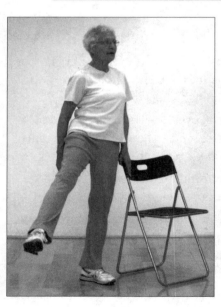

- Stand upright, with your feet together and with your shoulders over hips, hips over knees, and knees over ankles.

- Abduct (move outward, away from midline) your right leg.

- Hold this position for five to ten seconds before returning to the beginning position.

- Perform three to five repetitions, alternately.

- Initially, you may need to hold on to a sturdy object for balance. However, as you improve your balance with this exercise, keep both hands at your sides.

Knee Raise 🏠

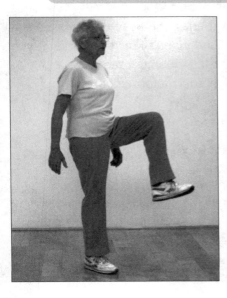

- Stand upright, with your feet together and with shoulders over hips, hips over knees, and knees over ankles.

- Flex your left hip, raising your knee to a point where your thigh is parallel to the floor.

- Hold this position for five to ten seconds.

- Perform three to five repetitions, alternately.

- Hold on to a sturdy object, if necessary.

Bosu Standing 🏠

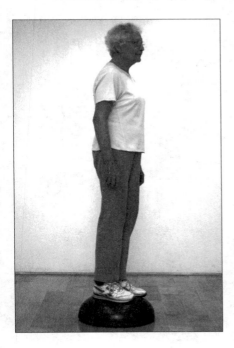

- On a Bosu, stand upright, with your feet two to three inches apart and with shoulders over hips, hips over knees, and knees over ankles.

- Hold this position for five to ten seconds.

- When standing on the Bosu is easy, increase your challenge by continuously stepping up and down from it, one foot at a time.

- Start by stepping up with the right foot, then the left foot.

- Pause, then step down first with the right, then the left foot.

- After twenty or thirty seconds of stepping, alternate the sequence by first stepping with the left foot, then with the right.

Note: There are a variety of devices designed to provide unstable surfaces, helping to challenge the neutralizers and stabilizers of the legs. One such device, Bosu, is pictured here. Of all the varieties, the Bosu was chosen as a starting point because it is neither extremely difficult nor too simple. If you choose to purchase the Bosu, it can also be used for other exercises—abs, legs, and upper body. (See Resources in back for product information).

Bosu Hip Flexion

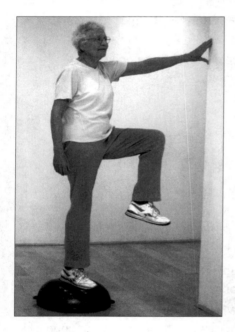

- On a Bosu, stand upright, with your feet two to three inches apart and with shoulders over hips, hips over knees, and knees over ankles.

- Flex your right hip, raising your knee to a point where your thigh is parallel to the floor.

- Hold this position for five to ten seconds.

- Perform three to five reps, alternately.

- Hold on to a sturdy object, if necessary.

16

Whole Body Workouts (for Beginners)

This chapter is devoted to beginners. Although the actual program setup is outlined in the next chapter, you will learn basic tips to get started in this chapter. The goal for this chapter is to encourage you to start, no matter how long it's been, if ever, since you last exercised. Thus, the language used is encouraging, positive, and non-judgmental. If you have exercise experience, you may skip this section and go directly to the *Program Options* section.

Getting Started—For the Absolute Beginner

Let's face it, you feel slower and more sluggish than you did when you were in your prime. Your body has aches in places you didn't have them before. You haven't moved in years and you're stiff. In fact, it's been so long, you just don't know how to break the mold of sitting on your glutes—whether in front of the TV or computer—every single night. Either this is an addiction, or it may simply be that you haven't noticed this is not how you're supposed to live your life. This simply is *not* living.

One major reason people avoid exercise is that they don't know how to take the first step—the most difficult step. Actually, the hardest part of any exercise program is just getting started, so let me take you through the basics to help make this part fun and easy. It's simpler than you think, and I will show you everything you need to know.

First of all, just be aware that you don't need to join an expensive gym. You don't need any of those fancy machines you see on TV, either. You don't even need much space in your home. All you really need is enough floor space to lie down on, an exercise mat, a Swiss ball, and some light weights. If space is too limited, there are adjustable dumbbells that require much less storage space. For example, instead of six separate pairs of dumbbells, you can have one pair that offers adjustments for six weight increments. With these dumbbells, you can pick and choose the appropriate exercises from the menus in Chapters 11–15. In Chapter 17, where program options are discussed, begin with the first choice. (Before beginning your routine, be sure to read Chapters 17 and 18.)

For as little as $205, the current price, you can have *all* the tools you'll need to start a thorough exercise routine. The Resources section in back lists places that will help you to find a mat, ball, and weights. Or, you may visit my website—www.ForzaFitness.com (click on Products)—for details on these items. (I hope this dispels the myth that it's too expensive to exercise—nothing could be further from the truth.)

If $205 is too much money, please don't think you're not ready to start yet. You are. Merely adjust what I'm saying to what you can afford. For instance, start with cans of soup instead of weights, and exercise on a rug in lieu of a mat. You can also buddy up with a partner and share the equipment I've suggested. Not only will it cost half as much, but also, working out with someone else can be twice as much fun.

What you wear when exercising matters, too—even if no one will see you. It is important that you dress appropriately for two reasons—comfort and commitment. Dressing properly helps contribute to what I call the psychology of success. When you dress the part, you become more committed, you tend to stay more focused. If you wear PJ's, you'll want to sleep or relax. If you're wearing street clothes, you'll want to go outside and do anything *but* exercise.

Also, in order to make exercise enjoyable, you must first feel comfortable. Loose-fitting clothes are ideal, preferably those made of materials that help the skin breathe or allow perspiration to be easily whisked away. Once again, check Resources in back, or my website, for clothing with the ideal fabrics.

Although it's been scientifically proven that exercise helps elevate mood, getting to that point is the tricky part. To help kick off each exercise session—and help bridge the gap between feeling good as a result of exercise and feeling good enough to *start* exercising—listen to music that can elevate your mood. Whether it's big band music, disco, salsa, or world music, choose the type that inspires you most, that makes you happiest and most energetic.

Another thing that's essential is privacy. You must do what it takes to avoid distractions. Find space that's separate from other people who aren't exercising and from potentially distracting objects—unread mail, magazines, and books. Other outside stimuli can be distracting as well. If an open window keeps causing you to look outside rather than exercise, close the blinds. Keep your answering-machine volume at its lowest level. No answering machine? Keep the phone off the hook. *Focus* is the key to success. Again, you only need a small amount of space. And in this space, you can do an entire workout using the few items I've suggested.

Whatever time of day you choose to exercise, try doing every session at that same time—the body functions best on consistent patterns of events (when you eat, exercise, sleep, etc.). Also, working out at the same time will allow you to more easily plan your meals (pre- and post-workout) and supplements efficiently, as covered in Chapter 5.

We're all creatures of habit. Whether you realize it or not, everyone quickly falls into routines. Why do you think TV shows are on at the same time every week? If you simply embrace the idea of adding a pre-set time to exercise into your daily schedule, be it morning, afternoon, or evening, you will soon see it is one habit you won't want to break.

And one more thing: As you begin to feel better about yourself, be sure to include aerobics in your routine, even if this just means taking a ten-minute walk, either outside or in your own living room. Walking briskly (back and forth) in your own home—or marching in place (in front of the TV)—is a simple way to start. Once you're comfortable with ten minutes—and you will sense a joy of movement as stress becomes diminished and your happy hormones kick in—then it will be easy to increase the duration to twenty minutes and more.

Putting It All Together

N ow that I have covered the underlying principles of fitness and nutrition and have detailed the the nuts and bolts of proper technique, it's time to put all the pieces of the fitness puzzle together. Randomly performing a series of separate, unconnected exercises is inefficient and even counterproductive— the same way that having all the parts to an unassembled bicycle with no assembly instructions would be. This chapter is about designing fitness routines—program options.

The previous six chapters presented numerous exercise options, demonstrating a variety of exercises for each major muscle group. Fear not. It is not intended for you to do them all in each workout. (If that were the case, then instead of lasting thirty to forty-five minutes, each workout would last about three to four days.) Those chapters, particularly Chapters 11–15, serve as menus. From those menus, you may pick and choose various blends of exercises.

Be aware, however, that not just any combination would be suitable. What is needed is the *right* combination of exercises working together in a proper sequence that yields the safest and most effective results. This sequencing is a major component for program options. A series of program options are offered to help accommodate your level of fitness, as well as your workout schedule. Additionally, there is a separate section devoted to people with various health problems (arthritis, bad knees, heart disease, low back pain, and so on).

Rules of Thumb

In order to optimally set up your routine, in terms of exercise sequencing and workout frequency, several principles need to be remembered when performing resistance-training routines. I'd like to reiterate that, for optimal results, cardio and resistance workouts need to be separate from each other. The body can only store a limited amount of energy. When both exercise modalities are performed back to back, benefits for each will be diminished. Ideally, they should be performed at different times of day, and enough time for rest and recovery (involving nutrient intake) should be allowed.

If, however, you have no choice but to perform both in the same workout, then to accomplish most goals (fat-burning, increased strength and balance, body sculpting, etc.), do the strength training first. There is only one condition under which you should do cardio training first, and that is if your primary goal is to enhance your cardiovascular capacity or aerobic functioning.

Now, for those rules of thumb.

- Always work larger muscles first, smaller muscles last. This is very important because larger muscles rely on smaller muscles for support. If you fatigue the smaller muscles first, then the larger ones won't be capable of handling the challenges they need to become stronger.

- Limit all strength-training workouts to no more than one hour and fifteen minutes. Hormonal changes (testosterone, cortisol) over this period of time make working out past seventy-five minutes suboptimal.

- Warm up prior to, and cool down following every workout. This translates to six to ten minutes of cardiovascular exercises involving steady *brisk* movement (cycle, rower, stepper, treadmill, etc.).

- If you choose to stretch prior to your workout, then do so only after thorough warm-ups (ten to twelve minutes of cardio). Also, avoid aggressive stretching and, instead, perform gentle core-area movements. Save your best, more vigorous stretches for the end of each respective muscle group's workout.

- Avoid working out the same muscle group two days in a row. Muscles require forty-eight hours to recover. If you're new to strength training, it is recommended that you work out every other day. As you advance, *split routines* may be applied, whereby you work out opposing muscles (pushing-vs-pulling muscle actions) on alternate days. To help you distinguish between opposing muscles of the upper body, the following chart illustrates the breakdown between pushing and pulling muscles.

Muscle actions are categorized under one of two possible motions: PUSHING or PULLING.

Pushing Muscle Groups	Pulling Muscle Groups
Chest (pectorals)	Back (latissimus dorsi)
Shoulders (deltoids)	Biceps
Triceps	

EXERCISE SEQUENCING MATTERS

The larger-to-smaller-muscles principle applies even within the scope of one particular muscle group. For example, when working your pecs (chest muscles), the optimal order for chest-pressing exercises is decline, flat, and incline press. The reason is, at the decline angle, you are working a larger band of muscle fibers than on the flat bench. At the decline, you are working the muscle fibers of the lower and mid pecs, and some fibers of the upper pecs as well. The flat bench version works a broader band of muscles than the incline angle. With the flat bench, fibers of the mid and upper pecs are used. For the incline press, only the upper-pec fibers (of all pec muscles) are activated, along with front delts. If you are on a tight schedule, always work the larger muscle groups, inasmuch as they will also recruit the smaller muscles for assistance.

PROGRAM OPTIONS

The following routines are broken down according to level of experience, but they are not the only options available. Rather, they are models of the most efficient designs to help you succesfully attain your goals. For each level (beginner, intermediate, and advanced), I have included two styles of routines. The first, labeled General Routine, simply lists the general breakdown of muscles to be exercised on different days of the week. The second style, labeled Specific Routine, lists sample exercises specific to the muscles to be challenged.

Please note that for each of the two styles, I incorporated the same exercises simply to illustrate how you can split them up into varying routines. For your own workouts, however, I recommend that you periodically choose different exercises for each respective muscle group. By periodically, I mean every six to eight weeks for beginners and four to six weeks for the more advanced. This is the amount of time it takes for the body to adapt to a given routine.

In the following charts, wherever the word *rest* is indicated, it pertains solely to rest from resistance training, not from all other forms of activity. On those days, it would be ideal to play sports (basketball, handball, tennis, volleyball, etc.) and/or perform aerobic activities (aerobic classes, bicycling, jogging, swimming, power walking, etc.). For aerobic exercising, feel free to perform with greater intensity and duration than on days of strength training.

Beginner Routine

If you're new to strength training, then a good way to begin is by performing one exercise per muscle group for the upper body (chest, back, shoulders, biceps, and triceps), two exercises for the lower body, and two for the abdominals. That's nine exercises total. This initial workout should last between twenty-five and thirty-five minutes.

Based on your initial strength level, it is ideal to work out two or three times a week. For first-time beginners, it is best to start with two times a week and have two or three days of rest between workouts. A basic breakdown of such a workout would be as follows.

Sample Workout Routine 1

General Routine

- Day 1: Lower body, upper body, core
- Day 2: Rest
- Day 3: Lower body, upper body, core
- Day 4: Rest
- Day 5: Lower body, upper body, core
- Days 6 and 7: Rest

Specific Routine

Monday	Tuesday	Wednesday	Thursday	Friday	Saturday	Sunday
Squats	**Rest**	Squats	**Rest**	Squats	**Rest**	**Rest**
Lunges		Lunges		Lunges		
Chest press		Chest press		Chest press		
Lat pulldown		Lat pulldown		Lat pulldown		
Shoulder press		Shoulder press		Shoulder press		
Biceps curl		Biceps curl		Biceps curl		
Tricep pressdown		Tricep pressdown		Tricep pressdown		
Core: Abdominals: -reverse crunch -obliques -crunch		**Core:** Abdominals: -reverse crunch -obliques -crunch		**Core:** Abdominals: -reverse crunch -obliques -crunch		
Back: -bridge extension		Back: -bridge extension		Back: -bridge extension		

For beginners, it's quite simple. Work out two to three times a week for two to four weeks. Each workout consists of one exercise per muscle group, for the entire body. Again, this translates into five exercises for the upper body: chest, back, shoulders, biceps, and triceps. For the lower body, begin with two exercises: squats and stationary lunges. If you belong to a gym and you have little balance, begin with the leg curl and leg extension machines.

The first two to six workouts should be strictly for introducing strength training to your body. So perform one set per exercise. After your body adapts to the initial shock of strength training, you should be ready to perform two sets per exercise. Some time after three or four weeks, begin introducing new exercises to your routine. Choose one new option from each muscle group's menu.

Intermediate Routines

As you become stronger and more familiar with resistance training, you can increase the intensity simply by splitting up your routine into separate workouts. In so doing, you will have more time to devote to each muscle. While there are many ways to perform split routines, a very simple way is to perform upper and lower body exercises on alternate days. The following is an example of such a split routine, a two-day split:

Sample Workout Routine 2

General Routine

- Day 1: Upper body
- Day 2: Lower body, abdominals
- Day 3: Rest
- Day 4: Upper body
- Day 5: Lower body, abdominals
- Days 6 and 7: Rest

Specific Routine

Monday	Tuesday	Wednesday	Thursday	Friday	Saturday	Sunday
Chest press	Squats	*Rest*	Chest press	Squats	*Rest*	*Rest*
Flyes	Lunges		Flyes	Lunges		
Lat pulldown	Leg curl		Lat pulldown	Leg curl		
Seated row	Leg extension		Seated row	Leg extension		
Shoulder press	Seated calf raise		Shoulder press	Seated calf raise		
Bicep curl	**Core:**		Bicep curl	**Core:**		
Tri pressdown	Abdominals:		Tri pressdown	Abdominals:		
	-reverse crunch			-reverse crunch		
	-obliques			-obliques		
	-crunch			-crunch		
	Back:			Back:		
	-bridge extension			-bridge extension		

Note: For the chest press, use either dumbbells or a machine.

Listed below is a bit more advanced program option. After trying the prior two choices for eight weeks each, you may want to consider progressing to the next routine. This one is good if you choose to work out your upper body two days in a row. It's designed in a way that separates the pulling and pushing muscles.

Sample Workout Routine 3

General Routine

- Day 1: Chest, shoulders, triceps
- Day 2: Back, biceps, core
- Day 3: Lower body
- Day 4: Chest, shoulders, triceps
- Day 5: Back, biceps, core
- Day 6: Lower body
- Day 7: Rest

Specific Routine

Monday	Tuesday	Wednesday	Thursday	Friday	Saturday	Sunday
Chest press	Lat pulldown	Squats	Chest press	Lat pulldown	Squats	*Rest*
DB incline press	Seated row	Lunges	Flyes	Seated row	Lunges	
Flyes	Standing low row	Leg curl	Lat pulldown	Standing low row	Leg curl	
Shoulder press	Standing curl twists	Leg extension	Seated row	Standing curl twists	Leg extension	
Cable rear deltoid	Concentrated curls	Squats	Shoulder press	Concentrated curls	Squats	
Tri pressdown (E-Z grip)		Seated calf raise	Bicep curl		Seated calf raise	
Rope tri pressdown	Core:	Anterior tibialis	Tri pressdown	Core:	Anterior tibialis	
	Abdominals:			Abdominals:		
	-reverse crunch			-reverse crunch		
	-toe taps			-toe taps		
	-obliques			-obliques		
	-ball crunch			-ball crunch		
	Back:			Back:		
	-bridge extension			-bridge extension		
	-prone limb raise			-prone limb raise		

Advanced Routines

Once your body has adapted to split routines, there are other ways to further challenge your strength levels at that point in time. Here are some examples.

Sample Workout Routine 4

General Routine

- Day 1: Back, triceps, core
- Day 2: Lower body
- Day 3: Chest, biceps, core
- Day 4: Rest
- Day 5: Shoulders, core
- Day 6: Lower body
- Day 7: Rest

Specific Routine

Monday	Tuesday	Wednesday	Thursday	Friday	Saturday	Sunday
Lat pulldown	Squats	Decline chest press	**Rest**	External rotation	Butt press	**Rest**
Standing rope pulldown	Lunges	Chest press		Rear deltoid	Adduction	
Seated row	Leg curl	Incline press		Shoulder press	Abduction	
Standing low row	Leg extension	Flyes		Cable internal rotation	Calf raise	
French press	Adduction	Concentrated curls			Anterior tibialis	
Cable kickbacks	Abduction	Standing curl twists				
V-tri pressdown		Hammer curls				

Core:	**Core:**	**Core:**
Abdominals:	Abdominals:	Abdominals:
-reverse crunch	-reverse crunch	-reverse crunch
-toe taps	-toe taps	-toe taps
-alternate obliques	-alternate obliques	-alternate obliques
-obliques	-obliques	-obliques
-ball obliques	-ball obliques	-ball obliques
-ball crunch	-ball crunch	-ball crunch
-crunch	-crunch	-crunch

Monday	Tuesday	Wednesday	Thursday	Friday	Saturday	Sunday
Back: -bridge extension -prone limb raise		Back: -bridge extension -prone limb raise		Back: -bridge extension -prone limb raise -hyperextension		

Sample Routine 5

General Routine

- Day 1: Back, core
- Day 2: Lower body
- Day 3: Chest, core
- Day 4: Rest
- Day 5: Shoulders, biceps, triceps
- Day 6: Lower body, core
- Day 7: Rest

Specific Routine

Monday	Tuesday	Wednesday	Thursday	Friday	Saturday	Sunday
Lat pulldown	Squats	Decline chest press	*Rest*	External rotation	Butt press	*Rest*
Standing rope pulldown	Lunges	Chest press		Rear deltoid	Adduction	
Seated row	Leg curl	Incline press		Shoulder press	Abduction	
Standing low row	Leg ext.	Pec deck		Concentrated curl	Calf raise	
Core: Abdominals: -reverse crunch -toe taps -alternate obliques -obliques -ball obliques -ball crunch -crunch		**Core:** Abdominals: -reverse crunch -toe taps -alternate obliques -obliques -ball obliques -ball crunch -crunch		Standing curl twists E-Z tri pressdown Rope tri pressdown	**Core:** Abdominals: -reverse crunch -toe taps -alternate obliques -obliques -ball obliques -ball crunch -crunch	

Monday	Tuesday	Wednesday	Thursday	Friday	Saturday	Sunday
Back: -bridge extension -prone limb raise		Back: -bridge extension -prone limb raise -hyperextension			Back: -bridge extension -prone limb raise	

Note: For the external rotation and rear deltoid exercises, you may choose either the dumbbell or cable variation, depending on which is available at your facility.

How Much Resistance?

Regarding the amount of resistance, I don't believe in playing around, using one and two pound weights forever. It's time to get serious. Even if you are over 150 years of age, you should avoid using toothpick-sized dumbbells—unless, of course, that is truly challenging for you by the tenth rep of a set. If you are younger than 150, I would recommend challenging your body to train just beyond what is comfortable, which would most likely be much more than one- and two-pounders.

In order for muscles to become stronger, they must be challenged just beyond their comfort zone—beyond what they're accustomed to handling. In other words, muscles need to be trained to momentary failure. We need to fatigue our muscles. It's the only way they will increase in strength. Generally speaking, an ideal resistance to work up to by your last set is 70–75 percent of your 1–RM, or 1 rep maximum (see Chapter 6 for more details). These percentages are estimates. If you are turned off by percentages, then more simply, remember that if you can perform a set of ten repetitions and feel muscular fatigue by the last three repetitions, you are challenging your muscles sufficiently. Therefore, the weight you used would be ideal for you.

Sets and Reps

The number of *sets* and *repetitions* (reps) you work with are important variables in designing your workout plan. A rep is one complete execution of an exercise, moving a resistance through a complete ROM, including both the upward and downward portions of that movement (see Chapter 9). A set consists of a series of reps performed consecutively. How many sets and reps you work with will determine the outcome of your exercise.

Here is a rough breakdown of how many sets should be performed per exercise, based on fitness level.

Fitness Level	Set Range
Beginner	1–2 sets
Intermediate	2–3 sets
Advanced	3–4 sets

The next question in your excited mind should be, "How many reps should be performed per set?" The answer depends on your intended outcome—your goals. For starters, the first set of each given muscle group should be considered a warm-up set. Therefore, always begin with a very light weight (35–40 percent of 1–RM) for fifteen repetitions, or a weight you could move fifteen times with little fatigue by the last repetition. For subsequent sets, use the following as a guideline for how many reps you should work with. (Also included in this chart are the suggested between-set rest intervals.)

Goals	Rep Range	Rest between sets
Muscle tone/trim down	10–12 reps	45–55 seconds
Strength increase/muscle growth	8–10 reps	55–75 seconds
Power increase	4–6 reps	3–4 minutes

The above rep ranges are not just arbitrary numbers to work toward, irrespective of resistance. Except for your warm-up sets, choose weight loads that bring on fatigue by the last three to four reps of each set. If you underestimated your strength level for a particular set, do not perform additional reps until you sense fatigue. Simply stop at the high end of your target rep range, rest for the appropriate interval, then increase the weight load according to how challenging (or unchallenging) the prior set was. Be sure to wear a watch with a second hand. How long you rest between sets is very important in successfully attaining your goals.

Modifications for Special Populations

If you have any health challenge, it is essential to first check with your doctor (provided she or he is thoroughly knowledgeable about exercise science) and a physical therapist, or exercise specialist, prior to beginning an exercise program. Here are some guidelines to consider for the following conditions.

Arthritis

Exercise is essential for preventing or managing arthritis. In general, exercise reduces joint pain and stiffness, increases the strength of muscle tissue surrounding the joints, and increases flexibility and endurance. Strength training is essential because strong muscles help lessen stress on the joints. Flexibility training is important in that such exercises help maintain proper range of motion, preventing the tightening of muscles and connective tissue.

For those with arthritis, both *isometric* and *isotonic* exercises are helpful. Experiment with each to find out which is more comfortable. For many people, the superior way to modify strength training, particularly on days when joints are inflamed, is to focus more on isometrics. Isometrics are the type of contractions that don't involve a movement of the joint. Isotonic exercises, on the other hand, involve joint movement during muscular contraction.

As for exercise in general, thorough cardio warm-ups and cool-downs are essential prior to and after all workouts for anyone with arthritis. In lieu of the standard six to ten minutes, I recommend ten to twelve minutes of cardio for this particular condition. Stretching exercises should follow both bouts of cardio. Strength-training frequency should not exceed three times per week.

Listen to your body. If any particular exercise causes discomfort, lighten the resistance, even if it's a resistance you've handled before. If persistent discomfort is experienced, shorten the duration of your session—as opposed to eliminating exercise entirely.

Asthma

Proper exercise programming can help control asthma, but one form, referred to as exercise-induced asthma, can also be triggered by exercise. While this is not a common problem during strength training or similar activities, there are several precautions to heed, particularly when performing brisk activities or exercising in colder environments. As with all forms of exercise, and particularly with special conditions, such as asthma, always perform adequate warm-up and cool-down exercises. This may mitigate exercise-induced asthma events. Drink plenty of water. Modify exercise intensity on days when you're more vulnerable to an asthma episode. Allow for more intense training on symptom-free days.

Diabetes

The primary concern for people with diabetes is to be aware of any potential drop in blood-sugar levels resulting from exercise. The timing of your pre-workout meals is critical. Also, be sure to have fruit juice and health snacks handy during your workout. If you sense any form of adverse insulin reactions (such as a lack of balance and coordination or disorientation), stop exercising immediately and sit down. Have a cup of juice and/or a healthy snack bar. As applies to all exercisers, people with diabetes need to drink sufficient fluids before, during, and after all workouts.

Frailty

Contrary to what most people realize, frailty occurs in both young and old people, although it naturally occurs more frequently in older people. A major cause for frailty is *sarcopenia,* or muscle loss, which is related to non-use. High-intensity resistance training is the only therapy that clearly demonstrates improvements in muscle loss. For frail individuals, the best way to begin a strength-training program safely is by performing only one set per exercise. Also, lighter resistances and fewer exercises should be applied. As strength begins to increase, the amount of resistance, the number of sets and the number of exercises should also be increased because the more strength training a frail person performs, the stronger he or she becomes.

Heart Disease

If you have cardiac problems, adhere to the guidelines provided by your physician. For post-coronary people, it is recommended to begin strength training at lighter loads, roughly in the range of 40 percent of your maximum resistance—or your 1–RM (see Chapter 6). Exercise in the higher rep range of twelve to fifteen reps. As you regenerate your strength and health, you may increase the intensity toward the 70–75 percent of 1–RM range, or the point where you can lift a weight for ten repetitions, feeling fatigue by the last three reps.

In lieu of working to fatigue on one exercise at a time, perform circuit training. Circuit training involves working a series of exercises in tandem. Avoid, or minimize, overhead pressing exercises (e.g., incline chest press, shoulder press). As with all exercising, but particularly for those with heart problems, always remember to breathe with each and every rep and avoid breath-holding as this places extra stress on the heart. Avoid *isometric* exercising, contractions that involve holding a resistance at one angle for several seconds at a time. If there are ever any signs of cardiovascular difficulties—abnormal heart rhythm, abnormal shortness of breath, chest discomfort, or dizziness—then cease exercising immediately.

Joint Injuries/Sensitivities

- **Knee.** Focus primarily on *closed-chain exercises* where your feet are planted on the floor or on a platform. Always be mindful of preventing your knees from passing your toes when performing pressing movements (butt press, lunges, squats, etc.). Thoroughly stretch your muscles after every workout and aerobic activity, particularly the hamstrings and quads—tight hamstrings and quads contribute to knee pain.

- **Shoulder** (*rotator cuff or bicipitus tendonitis*). Avoid overhead exercises. For the muscles of the back—lat pull-down and row exercises—avoid using straight-bar grips. Instead, use grips that allow your palms to face each other. For chest exercises, avoid using barbell free weights and barbell grips on machines. Use dumbbell free weights (they allow for modifications in positioning, providing more comfort and safety) and neutral, parallel grips on machines.

- **Elbow.** As with the shoulder, avoid using barbell free weights and barbell grips on machines.

- **Lower back.** The best way to strengthen the lower back is by challenging the core muscles (abs and lower back). However, if low back pain already exists, start light by performing only one or two exercises each session, and by doing fewer reps initially. Avoid overhead pressing movements. Be extra mindful of posture with all exercises—from doing stand-up bicep curls to laying-down chest presses, avoid overarching the lower back. If you have to cheat on form to squeeze out another rep, you'd be better off doing a *dropset*. A drop-set is when, midway through a set, you lower the resistance. This is safer for the back and it allows you to target your intended muscles more efficiently.

- **Neck.** Keep your neck muscles as relaxed as possible through all exercises. If you find yourself clenching your neck muscles, lighten the resistance. When performing chest exercises on the bench, avoid pressing your head into the bench as you press the weights upward.

Osteoporosis

Start your workout program with lighter weights—40–55 percent of your 1–RM. Over time, increase the resistance toward 70–80 percent 1–RM. Avoid overhead movements, such as the shoulder press.

If you have advanced stages of osteoporosis, then work out with lighter weights and work out on machines and benches that offer back and hip support. Avoid exercises that involve spinal flexion (bending) movements.

Sal's Summary

As important as it is to know exercises for each muscle group and understand the appropriate techniques relative to each exercise, it simply isn't enough to achieve success with your goals. It is critical to also know how to sequence your exercises and plan your workouts from one day to the next—this is like seeing the complete painting rather than just looking at each individual color. I urge you to avoid the mistake of exercising without a plan, but instead to follow a well-designed, smart approach to your fitness routine. You may have heard the popular adage on planning as it applies to other areas of life, such as business or education. Since it also applies here, in the world of health and fitness, I will reiterate that, *if you fail to plan, you are planning to fail.* So plan your workouts, and enjoy the fruits of your efforts—a stronger, leaner and, of course, more youthful YOU!

18

In a Nutshell

N ow the ball is in your court. I've laid the groundwork, so you can take the ball and move forward. In so doing, you must maintain a Positive Mental Attitude (PMA) in order to succeed with your fitness goals.

I once had a client who seemed to have made a conscious decision to forever hate exercise, and I sense he is representative of a huge percentage of the American population. See if he sounds at all familiar:

He arrived at the gym for each workout expressing (in a variety of ways) how much he despised exercise. After a workout, he always left the gym hating it. Even when we'd bump into each other on the street, he'd remind me how much he hated it. Not surprisingly, after several months of agonizing torture (for both of us), he dropped out and never returned. He did promise to find more enjoyable ways of getting fit, but five years later, his waistline has grown by five inches and he now gets winded walking along streets that have a slight incline.

The worst part about this client was that he did it to himself. He set himself up for failure from the start, before he ever stepped foot in the gym. Although he was able to intellectually understand the value of exercise, he was unable (or unwilling) to tap into his inner self and sense the power of exercise . . . the beauty of movement. His mind—his conscious decision to hate exercise— sabotaged all possibilities, all attempts to improve his well-being and his life overall.

On the other hand, I had a girlfriend who was determined to succeed. Overweight for a number of years and inactive for much of her life (her most vigorous activity was reading suspense novels), she woke up one day *tired* of always feeling tired. She knew in her heart that she was in control, and she was going to succeed in attaining a new figure and a new life simply through exercise and proper nutrition.

In a matter of eight weeks, she saw major changes occurring in her body, while simultaneously experiencing a heightened level of energy. Five years later, she is more active, more energetic, and more fit than she has ever been. Now, as a married couple, she and I support each other through moments of weakness—when the temptation occurs to have a doughnut or sit in front of the TV after dinner instead of going for our nightly walks.

What do these two stories have in common? Primarily my desire to change your views of going to the gym from negative to positive. During my twenty years as a fitness professional, a number of people have told me that working out in the gym is unnatural. Instead of thinking of it that way, however, recognize that what's truly unnatural for the body is the current environment we are all forced to live in.

Going to Dunkin' Donuts or McDonald's for food is unnatural. Having a Frapuccino is unnatural. Sitting in front of a TV for numerous hours every week is unnatural. Remember, the body is designed to be in motion. Also, in order to function optimally, the body needs to absorb a variety of minerals and nutrients—not chemicals put together in a lab to taste like food (read Eric Schlosser's *Fast Food Nation* and you'll see what I mean).

Going to the gym is not just good for the body, it's literally what the body *needs.* In today's society, people need to go out of their way to challenge their bodies. If you absolutely don't like the gym, then purchase resistance equipment for your home (you can e-mail me if you need help figuring out what is best for your space and budget). Don't let cost stand in your way. Today, there is something for almost all budgets. Start to view the weights and weight machines not as cold, frightening, foreign objects, but as warm friends with arms outstretched waiting to embrace you—friends who will help make you look and feel your best. Feel the interconnectedness between yourself and the metal as energy flows from you to the weights and back. (Metal is, after all, one of the major elements of our universe—it's part of our existence.)

If, at first, you just can't make yourself enjoy working out, then just *pretend* you do. After all, it's not as complicated or overwhelming as people imagine it to be. As I explained in Chapter 16, there is a very basic plan for newcomers—or returnees—to fitness. Just taking those first, tentative steps can often lead to an experience that becomes less and less difficult and more and more rewarding with each workout. With time, you'll begin to realize it not only makes you look and feel better, it also makes you think better—and it *will* ultimately save your life. Once you begin to feel, look, and think better, you will automatically come around to enjoying exercise more.

Taking it one step further, working out can become meditative. It has for me. This may sound a bit crazy, but if you think about it, meditation brings a deeper form of relaxation by helping you eliminate all the distractions of life, as well as the small, endless chatter going on in your mind.

When lifting weights, the ideal approach (for both safety and effectiveness) is to visualize—actually feel with your mind's eye—the exact muscles that need to be recruited for that particular movement. Too many times, people think about everything *but* the moment they are in. While lifting weights, they sometimes think about food, their spouse, or even not wanting to be there at the gym doing what they're doing. Big mistake.

As discussed in Chapter 9, by being in the moment, feeling each and every repetition, sensing the weight in your hands, taking deep breaths in as you lower the weight, and exhaling as you raise it back up, you will slowly become increasingly detached from the stressors of everyday life and more and more in tune with your core existence. And the more you do this, the stronger and more relaxed you will be. In fact, by the end of your workout, you will actually be generating a sense of ease and a heightened level of energy that is generally associated with meditation. One major difference, however, is that you will be more pumped (physically, mentally, and emotionally).

Hatred toward exercise is not only understandable, it's actually a common problem, usually due to a misconception about what's involved and how it should feel. It is really quite simple. Because, unfortunately, this is a society that offers far too many conveniences (thereby making everyone's lives more and more sedentary), it is essential to go out of your way and specifically schedule times for exercise and activity. If you've built barriers in your mind toward exercise, then change your mindset and come to terms with the *fact* that the human body—your body—needs movement, and lots of it.

Conclusion

E veryone interprets feeling good in different ways. Feeling *good* means so much more than simply not being sick, which is the usual definition of the term. What I have discovered is that feeling good is waking up in the morning energized and happy. It's being able to work a full day and still be vibrant and capable of enjoying activities during your free time or at night. It's when you are able to brush your hands over your body and honestly say, "Hey, I like how I feel—I feel GOOOOD!" There are chemical and hormonal changes that will help enlighten you emotionally and spiritually. And to think I used to connect exercise merely to the physical level. It is so much more. If you stick with it long enough, it will change your entire existence.

In addition to commenting about how I always seem energized, people around me also comment that I always look happy. This is one aspect of my appearance I literally never thought about previously. It simply never occurred to me. After all, I've had my share of hardships sprinkled throughout my life— from the bullies in elementary school to the heartbreaks in high school and later, plus debt, stress, occasional burnout, etc. Yet, through it all, exercise has helped me get—and stay—in touch with my inner self.

As I look back over my life, I realize what they say is true. I may have had a few downturns, but I have always bounced right back. And even during those gray moments in life, when I reach deep down inside, I realize I am, in fact, always happy. Wouldn't you be, too, if you felt stronger, healthier, and younger than in years past?

Trust me, there's nothing stopping you. Except, perhaps, yourself . . .

Following the principles and techniques laid out in *Stop Aging—Start Training* can help anyone regain and retain a high degree of youthfulness. All that is needed is patient effort applied consistently.

I'm certain you're already aware of books that promise the quick fix—results in ten minutes or less . . . per week. It's amazing how books continue to come out with a new method of exercise that somehow requires less time than was promised in any prior book, less time than it takes to eat ten grapes. I wouldn't be surprised if a book is currently being written on how to attain a healthy, fit body through just two minutes of exercises per week . . . visulaization exercises, that is.

There are two basic premises of human existence. The first is, ***the body was designed to absorb certain specific nutrients*** (and this does not include fast foods or junk foods—not even ice cream). The second premise—the one this book is built on—is that ***the body was designed to be in motion.*** If you honor these two laws of human nature, then you will live life to its fullest . . . in terms of longevity as well as health, vitality, and enthusiasm. So what are you waiting for? Start moving—start enjoying life to its fullest. Here's to the GOOD LIFE. *Stop Aging—Start Training!!!*

Glossary

Abs (abdominals). Muscles of the abdomen located between the diaphragm (attached to the rib cage) and the pelvis.

Absolute value. The value of a number without recognition of its relative worth.

Abductors. Muscles responsible for moving a body part (arm or leg) outward, away from the midline of the body.

Adaptation. The point at which a muscle is so used to an exercise that it no longer progresses from that activity.

Adductors. Muscles responsible for moving a body part (arm or leg) inward, toward the midline of the body.

Aerobic exercise. Low-intensity exercise that utilizes oxygen as the primary fuel source. Aerobics generally entail rhythmic movements that engage larger muscles at moderate levels of intensity for extended periods of time. Some examples include jogging, rope jumping, swimming, and walking.

Aerobic threshold. A heightened level of exercise intensity somewhat below the anaerobic threshold—the exercise is still considered aerobic.

Anabolism. The process of building up molecules, organs, and tissues. In the area of strength training, this translates to muscle growth.

Anaerobic exercise. Activities that are performed at a higher intensity level and are of a shorter duration than aerobic exercises. Lactic acid is a by-product of this type of exercise. Examples include sprinting and weightlifting.

Anaerobic threshold. The heightened level of exercise intensity at which lactic acid begins to accumulate (it is produced more quickly than it can be metabolized) in the blood. This is the point where you begin to switch over from aerobic to anaerobic metabolism.

Anterior tibialis. The muscle located on the front and lateral (outer) side of the shin bone (tibia); this muscle is responsible for raising your foot upward.

Antioxidants. Vitamin and food substances that aid in the removal of free-radical molecules that attack healthy cells in the body and leave the body vulnerable to cancer and other diseases.

Atherosclerosis. A disease of the arteries—the formation and accumulation of cholesterol-rich deposits, called plaque, on the inner lining of the arteries, leading to the narrowing and eventual closure of these vessels.

Back Extensors. Muscles positioned along both sides of the spine, extending the length of the back, that are responsible for straightening the torso and maintaining an upright position.

Biceps. Muscles on the front part of the upper arm responsible for flexing your arm, bringing your wrist closer to your shoulder; also responsible for turning your palm upward.

Cardiovascular conditioning. Exercise programs which enhance aerobic capacity, strengthening the heart and lungs, thereby enhancing your body's ability to deliver oxygen and other nutrients throughout the body.

Catabolism. The process of breaking down molecules, organs, and tissues. In the area of strength training, this translates to the breakdown of muscle tissue.

Cholesterol. A fat found in the bloodstream and in all the body's cells. Among other functions, it is used in the formation of cell membranes and some hormones. There is good (HDL) and bad (LDL) cholesterol. (A high level of total cholesterol and/or LDL cholesterol is a primary risk factor for heart disease.)

Complete protein. Foods that contain all the essential amino acids (building blocks). Of the twenty-two amino acids in a protein, nine cannot be manufactured by the body; those nine amino acids must be consumed through foods.

Core. Muscles in the central region of the body, including abdominals and back muscles, where all movement and balance originates.

Creeping obesity. The unobvious weight gain that occurs slowly, over time. The gain is so gradual it sometimes takes up to a decade to notice the changes that have been occurring.

Deltoids (delts). Triangular-shaped shoulder muscles primarily responsible for moving arms forward, backward, upward, and/or away from the body; they are divided into three main sections—anterior (front), posterior (rear), and medial.

Drop-set. Lowering the resistance to a lighter weight when reaching a state of fatigue during a particular exercise, so a few more repetitions will be completed for that set.

Ectomorph. A body type generally described as tall, slim, and angular.

Endomorph. A body type generally described as round and pear-shaped.

Energy balance. The net balance between calories consumed (through eating and drinking) and calories expended (through physical activity and biologic functioning).

Erector spinae. *See Back extensors.*

Essential amino acids. The nine amino acids (building blocks) the body is not capable of producing, that must be absorbed through food.

Essential body fat. The amount of body fat necessary for normal body functioning; for men, this is in the 3–5 percent range, while for women, the range is 8–10 percent.

E-Z barbell. A barbell with grips shaped like an E and a Z; these help ease the potential pressure on wrists that can occur with straight barbells.

Glycemic index. A measure of how high blood sugar rises in response to the consumption of fifty grams of carbohydrates of a particular food.

Glycemic load. A representation of how much blood sugar is in the body, for the body to handle over time. This is determined by multiplying a glycemic-index value of a food by the quantity of the food being measured.

Ground reaction forces. The reaction force supplied by the ground, through the body, in relation to the amount of force exerted by the body onto the ground.

Heart-rate monitor. A device that measures your heart rate at any given moment. The more accurate models have two components: a chest-strap transmitter and a wristwatch receiver.

Hemoglobin. A complex molecule found in red blood cells, which contains iron and protein; it transports oxygen from the lungs to the rest of the body, including the muscles.

Hydrostatic (underwater) weighing. A method of measuring body-fat percentage, whereby the person is completely submerged in water and the weight underwater is compared with her or his weight in air. This is considered the gold standard of body-fat measurement; lab equipment and technicians are needed.

Incomplete protein. A food that lacks, or is low in, one or more of the nine essential amino acids.

Isometrics. A form of exercise during which there is no change at a joint angle, or in the length of a muscle, as tension is applied.

Isotonics. A form of exercise during which the joint angle changes, as does the muscle's length.

Kinesiology. The study of body movement and the causes and consequences of physical activity.

Macronutrient. The nutrients needed to provide the body and brain with the energy necessary to maintain basic functions at rest and during physical activity. There are three categories: carbohydrates, fat, and protein.

Maximal heart rate. The maximum heart rate a person should achieve during maximal physical exertion. Although there are many formulas, the most common measure for determining this is to subtract your age from 220. One other measure, which is slightly less conservative, is to subtract one half of your age from 210.

Mesomorph. The body type generally described as athletic, muscular, and broad-shouldered—hourglass-shaped for women and rectangular-shaped for men. This category is mid-range between ectomorph and endomorph.

Micronutrients. Vitamins and minerals that have highly specific roles in facilitating energy transfer and tissue synthesis. Unlike macronutrients, these are needed in relatively small quantities. The most beneficial types are those acquired through table foods. For those difficult to acquire through foods, supplements are helpful, if not essential.

Midline. An imaginary line going down the center of the body, separating the left from the right side.

Multifidus. Muscles deep in the spine, on either side of the vertebrae, that assist the erector spinae in keeping the spine erect and able to rotate.

Muscular endurance. The ability of a muscle, or muscle group, to perform repeated contractions against a light resistance for an extended period of time.

Neutralizers. Secondary support muscles that assist primary muscle movers by helping maintain balance and stability.

Overload. Applying progressively more resistance to a muscle than that muscle is used to handling.

Phytochemicals. Antioxidants and other nutrients contained in fruits and vegetables.

Relative value. The value of a number while recognizing its worth in relation to other variables.

Repetition (rep). One complete movement of an exercise through both upward and downward motions.

Sarcopenia. The age-related loss of muscle tissue and resulting loss of strength and function.

Saturated fat. The type of fat that is usually hardened at room temperature (butter, lard, and cream are some examples); these fats more readily block arteries, leading to heart disease.

Set. One group of consecutive repetitions of an exercise performed continuously without stopping.

Shock the body. This has nothing to do with electricity. It involves the introduction of a new exercise or routine to which the body has not yet adapted.

Sit and reach test. A flexibility test that primarily measures the range of motion of the back and hamstrings.

Somatotyping. The visual appraisal of body types—there are generally three: thin (ectomorph), medium build (mesomorph), and heavy (endomorph).

Spot reducing. The false notion that the body can lose fat in specific locations upon will.

Stabilizers. Muscles which support the movement of primary muscles, helping to maintain equilibrium and balance.

Stress test. A graded exercise test designed to evaluate the body's physiological responses to progressive demands, measured through the use of an EKG (electrocardiogram); such tests can be performed using either a bicycle ergometer or a motor-driven treadmill.

Submaximal stress test. A stress test that has the person peak out at a predetermined level of intensity, which is lower than his or her maximal capacity for exercise.

Superset. A training technique in which the exerciser performs one round of two or more consecutive exercises prior to resting.

Target heart-rate range. A predetermined heart-rate range to strive for, and maintain, during exercise; formulas are based on age.

Tendonitis. Inflammation of a tendon (the point where a muscle attaches to bone).

Triglycerides. A form of fat in the bloodstream. People with high triglycerides tend to have high total cholesterol, high LDL (bad) cholesterol and low HDL (good) cholesterol level. A high triglyceride level is associated with heart disease.

Waist-to-hip ratio. A simple, effective measure of fat distribution. To gauge the proportion of fat stored around your waist and hips, divide the circumference of your waist (the smallest section of your waist) by the circumference of your hips (the widest part of your buttocks). See Chapter 6 for more information.

Warm-up, general. A light intensity of exercise performed to literally warm up the body by elevating the core temperature, gradually raising the heart rate to a working level, and preparing the joints for more intense activity. An excellent method for general warm-ups is light, brisk aerobic exercise—examples include brisk walking and slow cycling.

Warm-up, specific. A lighter version of exercise which mimics, or uses the same muscles as, the activity or exercise about to be engaged in; exercise with a weight/resistance that is roughly 50% of your strength capacity for that particular exercise.

Resources

Adjustable Dumbbells

Power Block

1071 32nd Ave NW
Owatonna, MN 55060
Ph: 1-507-451-5152
Fax: 1-507-451-5278
Website: www.powerblock.com
e-mail: questions@powerblock.com

This company specializes in the Power Block dumbbells and accessories, including benches and dumbbell racks. They also offer a home gym.

Versa-Bell

Although no specific manufacturer is given, there are many places listed on the Internet that sell these dumbbells, including Amazon.com, Walmart.com, and Yahoo.com.

Bowflex SelectTech

Ph: 1-800-850-3280 or
  1-800-269-3539
Website: www.bowflexselecttech.
  com
e-mail: customerservice@bowflex.
  com

This company offers adjustable dumbbells as well as a strength-conditioning home gym, a cardio apparatus and workout accessories.

Balance and Resistance Devices

Bosu Balance Trainer
Team Bosu
1400 Raff Road
Canton, OH 44750
Ph: Toll free: 1-800-321-9236
Website: www.bosu.com

This company supplies the Bosu balance exercise tool along with instructional videos.

Dyna-Band
Crown World Marketing
PO Box 1195
Naphill, High Wycombe
Buckinghamshire HP14 4WQ
United Kingdom
Ph: + 44 (0) 870 9504133
Fax: + 44 (0) 870 9504134
Website: www.dynaband.co.uk
e-mail: info@dynaband.co.uk,
    sales@dynaband.co.uk

This company supplies resistance bands in a series of intensities.

Thera-Band
The Hygenic Corporation
1245 Home Avenue
Akron, OH 44310
Ph: 1-800-321-2135
Fax: 1-330-633-9359
Website: www.thera-band.com
e-mail: feedback@hygenic.com

This company offers a variety of exercise products, including balance devices, resistance bands, and stability balls. They also offer a number of aquatic accessories, including buoyancy and resistance devices.

Exercise Mats and Stability Balls

Aeromat Fitness Products
2070 Zankar Road
San Jose, CA 95131
Ph: 1-877-278-6158
Fax: 1-707-221-4040
Website: www.aeromats.com
e-mail: info@aeromats.com

This company offers a variety of exercise tools, including mats, stability balls, weighted resistance balls, and balance devices.

Airex Exercise Mats
Although no specific manufacturer is given, there are many places listed on the Internet that sell these mats, including Amazon.com. Two companies I have purchased exercise equipment from are Perform Better and Power Systems, listed below.

SPRI Products, Inc.
1600 Northwind Blvd.
Libertyville, IL 60048
Ph: 1-800-222-7774
Website: www.spriproducts.com
e-mail: teamspri@spriproducts.com

This company designs, manufactures, and distributes rubberized resistance exercise products.

Perform Better, Inc
M-F Athletic Company
P.O. Box 8090
Cranston, RI 02920-0090
Ph: 1-888-556-7464 or
    1-401-942-9363
Fax: 1-800-682-6950
Website: www.performbetter.com
e-mail: performbetter@mfathletic.
    com

This company specializes in athletic equipment, including exercise mats and stability balls, balance devices, resistance bands, and learning tools (books, DVDs, and videos).

Power Systems, Inc.
P.O. Box 31709
Knoxville, TN 37930
Ph: 1-800-321-6975 or
    1-865-769-8223
Fax: 1-800-298-2057 or
    1-865-769-8211
Website: www.power-systems.com
e-mail: customerservice@
    power-systems.com

This company is a distributor for a variety of fitness and sports products, including exercise mats, stability balls, balance devices, resistance bands, and learning tools (books, DVDs, and videos).

Exercise Benches

Reebok Step Bench
FreeMotion Fitness
1096 Elkton Drive, Suite 600
Colorado Springs, CO 80907
Ph: 1-877-363-8449 or
    1-719-955-1100
Fax: 1-719-955-1104
Website: www.freemotionfitness.com
e-mail: customerservice@
    freemotion fitness.com

This company, a subsidiary of ICON Health and Fitness, manufactures and markets step benches and other aerobic and resistance equipment.

JP Design and Manufacturing, Inc.
106 Shelbourne Drive
York, PA 17403
Ph: 1-866-917-8776 or
    1-717-854-1668
Fax: 1-717-846-8200
Website: www.jpdesignandmfg.com
e-mail: jpdesign@jpdesignandmfg.
    com

This company, which manufactures therapeutic and exercise equipment, has a weightlifting bench that is both portable and adjustable.

Organizations

American College of Sports Medicine (ACSM)
P.O. Box 1440
Indianapolis, IN 46206-1440
Ph: 1-317-637-9200
Fax: 1-317-634-7817
Website: www.acsm.org.
e-mail: membership@acsm.org

This association certifies fitness trainers and exercise physiologists and promotes fitness, health, and quality of life through research and education.

American Council on Exercise (ACE)
4851 Paramount Drive
San Diego, CA 92123
Ph: 1-888-825-3636 or
    1-858-279-8227
Fax: 1-858-279-8064
Website: www.acefitness.org.
e-mail: support@acefitness.org

This association certifies fitness trainers and promotes quality of life through research on safe and effective physical activity.

National Strength and Conditioning Association (NSCA)
1885 Bob Johnson Drive
Colorado Springs, CO 80906
Ph: 1-800-815-6826 or
    1-719-632-6722
Fax: 1-719-632-6367
Website: www.nsca-lift.org
e-mail: nsca@nsca-lift.org

This association certifies fitness trainers as well as strength and conditioning specialists for sports and disseminates research-based information to improve athletic performance and fitness.

In addition to the companies/manufacturers listed, you may also do an Internet search to find a variety of distributors offering the same products at competitive prices.

References

Chapter 3

Ades, PA, DL Ballor, T Ashikaga, et al. "Weight training improves walking endurance in healthy elderly persons." *Annals of Internal Medicine.* 124(6):568–572, 1996.

Ades, PA, PD Savage, M Brochu, et al. "Resistance training increases total daily energy expenditure in disabled older women with coronary heart disease." *Journal of Applied Physiology.* 98(4):1280–1285, 2005.

Andrews, GR. "Care of older people: Promoting health and function in an ageing population." *British Medical Journal.* 322:728–729, 2001.

Bemben, DA, NL Fetters, MG Bemben, et al. "Musculoskeletal responses to high- and low-intensity resistance training in early postmenopausal women." *Medicine and Science in Sports and Exercise.* 32(11):1949–1957, 2000.

Beniamini, Y, JJ Rubenstein, AD Faigenbaum, et al. "High-intensity strength training of patients enrolled in an outpatient cardiac rehabilitation program." *Journal of Cardiopulmonary Rehabilitation.* 19(1):8–17, 1999.

Beniamini, Y, JJ Rubenstein, LD Zaichkowsky, et al. "Effects of high-intensity strength training on quality-of-life parameters in cardiac rehabilitation patients." *American Journal of Cardiology.* 80(7):841–846, 1997.

Blain, H, A Vuillemin, A Teissier, et al. "Influence of muscle strength and body weight and composition on regional bone mineral density in healthy women aged sixty years and over." *Gerontology.* 47(4):207–212, 2001.

Brochu, M, P Savage, M Lee, et al." Effects of resistance training on physical function in older disabled women with coronary heart disease." *Journal of Applied Physiology.* 92:672–678, 2002.

Bronder, D, R Lorenz, JK Schneider. "Is exercise behavior related to positive subjective feelings in older adults?" *Medicine and Science in Sports and Exercise.* 36(5):S48, 2004.

Castaneda, C, JE Layne, L Munoz-Orians, et al. "A randomized controlled trial of resistance exercise training to improve glycemic control in older adults with type 2 diabetes." *Diabetes Care.* 25:2335–2341, 2002.

Cononie, CC, JE Graves, ML Pollock, et al." Effect of exercise training on blood pressure in seventy- to seventy-nine-year-old men and women." *Medicine and Science in Sports and Exercise.* 23(4):505–511, 1991.

Daub, WD, GP Knapik, WR Black. "Strength training early after myocardial infarction." *Journal of Cardiopulmonary Rehabilitation.* 16(2):100–108, 1996.

Doherty, TJ. "Physiology of Aging – Invited Review: Aging and sarcopenia." *Journal of Applied Physiology.* 95:1717–1727, 2003.

Downey, WJ, JA Chromiak, JM Hood, et al. "Effect of a post-exercise recovery supplement and ten-week strength training program on muscle strength and endurance." *Medicine and Science in Sports and Exercise.* 36(5):S42, 2004.

Dunstan, DW, RM Daly, N Owen, et al. "High-intensity resistance training improves glycemic control in older patients with type 2 diabetes." *Diabetes Care* 25:1729–1736, 2002.

Elliott, KJ, C Sale, NT Cable. "Effects of resistance training and detraining on muscle strength and blood lipid profiles in postmenopausal women." *British Journal of Sports Medicine.* 36:340–344, 2002.

Fagard, RH. "Impact of different sports and training on cardiac structure and function." *Cardiology Clinics.* 15(3):397–412, 1997.

Fatouros, IG, K Taxildaris, SP Tokmakidis, et al. "The effects of strength training, cardiovascular training and their combination on flexibility of inactive older adults." *International Journal of Sports Medicine.* 23:112–119, 2002.

Feigenbaum, MS, ML Pollock. "Prescription of resistance training for health and disease." *Medicine and Science in Sports and Exercise.* 31(1):38–45, 1999.

Fiatarone, MA, EC Marks, ND Ryan, et al. "High-intensity strength training in nonagenarians. Effects on skeletal muscle." *Journal of the American Medical Association (JAMA).* 263(22), 1990.

Gauchard, GC, A Tessier, C Jeandel, et al. "Improved muscle strength and power in elderly exercising regularly." *International Journal of Sports Medicine.* 24:71–74, 2003.

Ghilarducci, LE, RG Holly, EA Amsterdam. "Effects of high resistance training in coronary artery disease." *American Journal of Cardiology.* 64(14):866–870, 1989.

Goldberg L, DL Elliot, RW Schutz, et al. "Changes in lipid and lipoprotein levels after weight training." *Journal of the American Medical Association (JAMA).* 252(4):504–506, 1984.

Holm, L, JL Olesen, P Schwarz, et al. "Enhanced musculoskeletal adaptation to resistance exercise training when nutrients are ingested immediately after training." *Medicine and Science in Sports and Exercise.* 36(5):S42, 2004.

Honkola, A, T Forsen, J Eriksson. "Resistance training improves the metabolic profile in individuals with type 2 diabetes." *Acta Diabetologica.* 34(4):245–248, 1997.

Hurley, BF, JM Hagberg, AP Goldberg, et al." Resistive training can reduce coronary risk factors without altering VO2max or percent body fat." *Medicine and Science in Sports and Exercise.* 20(2):150–154, 1988.

Hurley, BF, SM Roth. "Strength training in the elderly: effects on risk factors for age-related diseases." *Sports Medicine.* 30(4):249–268, 2000.

Kanakis, C, RC Hickson. "Left ventricular responses to a program of lower-limb strength training." *Chest.* 78:618–621, 1980.

Kelley, GA, KS Kelley. "A Meta-Analysis of Randomized Controlled Trials." *Hypertension.* 35:838, 2000.

Kraemer, WJ, K Adams, E Cafarelli, et al. "Progression models in resistance training for healthy adults—Position Stand." *Medicine and Science in Sports and Exercise.* 34(2):364–380, 2002.

Martel, GF, DE Hurlbut, ME Lott, et al. "Strength training normalizes resting blood pressure in sixty-five- to seventy-three-year-old men and women with high normal blood pressure." *Journal of the American Geriatric Society.* 47(10):1215–1221, 1999.

McCartney, N. "Role of resistance training in heart disease." *Medicine and Science in Sports and Exercise.* 30(10 Suppl):S396–402, 1998.

Miura, H, E Nakagawa, S Aoki, et al. "Effects of low-intensity resistance training on large artery stiffness in elderly men." *Medicine and Science in Sports and Exercise.* 36(5):S50, 2004.

Nelson, ME, MA Fiatarone, CM Morganti, et al. "Effects of high-intensity strength training on multiple risk factors for osteoporotic fractures. A randomized controlled trial." *Journal of the American Medical Association (JAMA).* 272(24), 1994.

Perrig-Chiello, P, WJ Perrig, R Ehrsam, et al. "The effects of resistance training on well-being and memory in elderly volunteers." *Age and Ageing.* 27:469–475, 1998.

Reeves, ND, CN Maganaris, MV Narici. "Effect of strength training on human patella tendon mechanical properties of older individuals." *Journal of Physiology.* 548(3): 971–981, 2003.

Rhea, MR, BA Alvar, LN Burkett, et al. A meta-analysis to determine the dose response for strength development. *Medicine and Science in Sports and Exercise.* 35(3):456–464, 2003.

Roberts, CK, RJ Barnard. "Effects of exercise and diet on chronic disease." *Journal of Applied Physiology.* 98:3–30, 2005.

Rogers, MA, WJ Evans. "Changes in skeletal muscle with aging: effects of exercise training." *Exercise and Sport Sciences Review.* 21:65-102, 1993.

Schilke, JM, GO Johnson, TJ Housh, et al. "Effects of muscle-strength training on the functional status of patients with osteoarthritis of the knee joint." *Nursing Research.* 45(2):68–72, 1996.

Schmitz, KH, RL Ahmed, D Yee. "Effects of a nine-month strength training intervention on insulin, insulin-like growth factor (IGF)-I, IGF-binding protein (IGFBP)-1, and IGFBP-3 in 30–50-year-old women." *Cancer Epidemiology, Biomarkers and Prevention.* 11:1597–1604, 2002.

Sipila, S, H. Suominen. "Effects of strength and endurance training on thigh and leg muscle mass and composition in elderly women." *Journal of Applied Physiology.* 78:334–340, 1995.

Spruit, MA, R Gosselink, T Troosters, et al. Resistance *versus* endurance training in patients with COPD and peripheral muscle." *European Respiratory Journal.* 19:1072–1078, 2002.

Stewart, KJ, LD McFarland, JJ Weinhofer, et al. "Safety and efficacy of weight training soon after acute myocardial infarction." *Journal of Cardiopulmonary Rehabilitation.* 18(1):37–44, 1998.

Tanasescu, M, MF Leitzmann, EB Rimm, et al. Exercise type and intensity in relation to coronary heart disease in men. *Journal of the American Medical Association (JAMA).* 288(16):1994–2000, 2002.

Tucker, LA, K Maxwell. "Effects of weight training on the emotional well-being and body image of females: predictors of greatest benefit." *American Journal of Health Promotion.* 6(5):338-344, 371, 1992.

Tucker, LA, LJ Silvester. "Strength training and hypercholesterolemia: an epidemiologic study of 8499 employed men." *American Journal of Health Promotion.* 11(1): 35–41, 1996.

Ullrich, IH, CM Reid, RA Yeater. "Increased HDL-cholesterol levels with a weight lifting program." *Southern Medical Journal.* 80(3):328–331, 1987.

Willardson, JM. "Sarcopenia and Exercise: Mechanisms, interactions, and application of research findings." *Strength and Conditioning Journal.* 26(6):26–31, 2004.

Winett, RA, RN Carpinell. "Potential health-related benefits of resistance training." *Preventive Medicine.* 33(5):503–513, 2001.

Wolfe, BL, LM LeMura, PJ Cole. "Quantitative analysis of single- vs. multiple-set programs in resistance training." *The Journal of Strength and Conditioning Research.* 18(1):35–47, 2004.

Zacker, RJ. "Strength Training in Diabetes Management." *Diabetes Spectrum.* 18: 71–75, 2005.

Chapter 5

Baechle, TR. *Essentials of Strength Training and Conditioning.* Champaign, IL: Human Kinetics. 1994.

Balch, JF, PA Balch. *Prescription for Nutritional Healing.* Garden City Park, NY: Avery Publishing Group. 1997.

Goldberg, DP, A Gitomer, R Abel. *The Best Supplements For Your Health*. New York, NY: Kensington Publishing Corp., 2002.

Kirschmann, GJ, JD Kirschmann. *Nutrition Almanac (4th Edition)*. New York, NY: McGraw-Hill, 1996.

McArdle, WD, FI Katch, VL Katch. *Exercise Physiology (4th Edition)*. Baltimore, MD: Williams and Wilkins, 1996.

Shintani, T. *The Good Carbohydrate Revolution*. New York, NY: Pocket Books, 2002.

Chapter 6

American College of Sports Medicine. *ACSM's Guidelines for Exercise Testing and Prescription (5th Edition)*. Media, PA: Williams and Wilkins, 1995.

Baechle, TR. *Essentials of Strength Training and Conditioning*. Champaign, IL: Human Kinetics. 1994.

Dos-Santos, JE, KS Oths, WW Dressler. "Socioeconomic factors and adult body composition in a developing society." *Revista Brasileira Hipertensao (Brazilian Journal of Hypertension)*. 8:173–178, 2001.

Freedman, DS, AA Rimm. "The relation of body fat distribution, as assessed by six girth measurements, to diabetes mellitus in women." *American Journal of Public Health*. 79(6):715–720, 1989.

Hartz, AJ, DC Rupley, AA Rimm. "The association of girth measurements with disease in 32,856 women." *American Journal of Epidemiology*. 119(1):71–180, 1984.

McArdle, WD, FI Katch, VL Katch. *Exercise Physiology (4th Edition)*. Baltimore, MD: Williams and Wilkins, 1996.

Norgan, NG. "The beneficial effects of body fat and adipose tissue in humans." *International Journal of Obesity and Related Metabolic Disorders*. 21(9):738–746, 1997.

Prentice, AM, and SA Jebb. "Beyond body mass index." *Obesity Review*. 2(3):141–147, 2001.

Chapter 7

Baechle, TR. *Essentials of Strength Training and Conditioning*. Champaign, IL: Human Kinetics, 1994.

Bonaiuti, D, B Shea, R Iovine, et al. "Exercise for preventing and treating osteoporosis in postmenopausal women." *Evidence-Based Nursing*. 6(2):50–51, 2003.

Bus, SA. "Ground reaction forces and kinematics in distance running in older-aged men." *Medicine and Science in Sports and Exercise*. 35(7):1167-1175, 2003.

DeSouza, CA, LF Shapiro, CM Clevenger, et al. "Regular aerobic exercise prevents and restores age-related declines in endothelium-dependent vasodilation in healthy men." *Circulation*. 102(12):1351–1357, 2000.

Fagard, RH. "The role of exercise in blood pressure control: supportive evidence." *Journal of Hypertension.* 13(11):1223-1227, 1995.

Farrell, SW, JB Kampert, HW Kohl, et al. "Influences of cardiorespiratory fitness levels and other predictors on cardiovascular disease mortality in men." *Medicine and Science in Sports and Exercise.* 30(6):899-905, 1998.

Friedenreich, CM, MR Orenstein. "Physical activity and cancer prevention: etiologic evidence and biological mechanisms." *Journal of Nutrition.* 132(11 Suppl):3456S–3464S, 2002.

Halbert, JA, CA Silagy, P Finucane, et al. "The effectiveness of exercise training in lowering blood pressure: a meta-analysis of randomised controlled trials of four weeks or longer." *Journal of Human Hypertension.* 11(10):641–649, 1997.

Kemmler, W, K Engelke, J Weineck, et al. "The Erlangen fitness osteoporosis prevention study: a controlled exercise trial in early postmenopausal women with low bone density-first-year results." *Archives of Physical Medicine and Rehabilitation.* 84(5): 673–682, 2003.

Kokkinos, PF, P Narayan, JA Colleran, et al. "Effects of regular exercise on blood pressure and left ventricular hypertrophy in African-American men with severe hypertension." *New England Journal of Medicine.* 333(22):1462–1467, 1995.

Luscher, TF, FC Tanner, MR Tschudi, et al. "Endothelial dysfunction in coronary artery disease." *Annual Review of Medicine.* 44:395-418, 1993.

Sturm, B, M Quittan, GF Wiesinger, et al. "Moderate-intensity exercise training with elements of step aerobics in patients with severe chronic heart failure." *Archives of Physical Medicine and Rehabilitation.* 80(7):746–750, 1999.

Thompson, PD, D Buchner, IL Piña, et al. "Exercise and physical activity in the prevention and treatment of atherosclerotic cardiovascular disease." *Circulation.* 107 (24):3109–3116, 2003.

Wei, M, LW Gibbons, TL Mitchell, et al. "The association between cardiorespiratory fitness and impaired fasting glucose and type 2 diabetes mellitus in men." *Annals of Internal Medicine.* 130(2):89–96, 1999.

Whelton, SP, A Chin, X Xin, et al. "Effect of aerobic exercise on blood pressure: a meta-analysis of randomized, controlled trials." *Annals of Internal Medicine.* 136 (7):493–503, 2002.

Chapter 17

Cotton, RT, RE Andersen. *Clinical Exercise Specialist Manual.* San Diego, CA: American Council on Exercise, 1999.

Westcott, WL, TR Baechle. *Strength Training for Seniors.* Champaign, IL: Human Kinetics, 1999.

Recommended Reading

Baechle, TR. *Essentials of Strength Training and Conditioning.* Champaign, IL: Human Kinetics. 1994.

Barnard, N. *The Power of Your Plate.* Summertown, TN: Book Publishing Company. 1995.

Goldberg, DP, A Gitomer, R Abel. *The Best Supplements For Your Health.* New York, NY: Kensington Publishing Corp., 2002.

Jensen, B, M Anderson. *Empty Harvest.* Garden City Park, NY: Avery Publishing Group, Inc. 1995.

Kirschmann, GJ, JD Kirschmann. *Nutrition Almanac, 4th edition.* New York, NY: McGraw-Hill. 1996.

Robbins, J. *Diet For A New America.* Tiburon, CA: HJ Kramer, Inc, 1998.

Schlosser, E. *Fast Food Nation.* New York, NY: Perennial, 2002.

Shintani, T. *The Good Carbohydrate Revolution.* New York, NY: Pocket Books, 2002.

Index

About the Models

Paul Auerbach

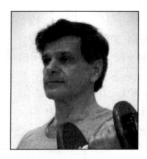

Exercising is one of the vital and defining habits of my life. Along with my efforts to eat properly, exercise has enabled me to continue to feel energetic and healthy. Prior to my retirement last year (as a high school teacher of incarcerated adolescents), my time at the gym was very important in helping me relieve stress. I continue to enjoy myself at the gym and am deeply grateful for the feeling of well-being it brings. The camaraderie gained from the gym has also been a nice addition to my life.

During the warmer months of the year, I add bike riding to my health regimen. I ride about 30 miles on each of the three days per week I bike on the trails of Long Island. At 63 years of age, I am very thankful that I can still experience the sense of physical exhilaration and healthiness that results from exercising.

Carmela Fichera

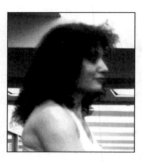

I've been active all of my life but started exercising at a gym since the age of 26. Now, at the age of 49, I've been a gym member for 23 years. Exercise has given me a lot of muscle tone. I feel and look younger and stronger. I notice I require less sleep and have great energy and endurance. In spite of my daily 2.5 hour commute (each way) of going to work, I that find exercise sustains me. I actually enjoy working out because it relieves so much stress. Exercise actually gives me the feeling of being on top of the world!

Irini Res

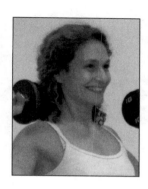

As a Jazz vocalist, Yoga, and Ballet teacher, I find exercising to be my source of physical, mental, and emotional energy. Exercising enables me—a woman in her sixth decade of life—to participate in these art forms with strength, stamina, and confidence. Exercising also provides me with energy and a positive outlook. This feeling—a heightened sense of well being—enables me to maintain my rigorous schedule. For me, everything flows from exercising.

Katherine Fichera

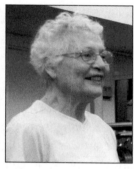

I was born with a passion for physical activity. I always felt energetic, happy, and healthy whenever I was in motion. Whether on the tennis court, the handball court, the roller rink, or the dance floor—it has given me continual strength. With only three to four hours of sleep, sports helped me cope with stress, responsibilities, and negativity. Working out is what gives me the strength and agility to be active.

As I look around, I see myself looking stronger, more energetic, and healthier than people half my age thanks to all the activities I have done throughout my life time. I am now 76 years old and my future goals are to exercise and play sports—the loves of my life (second to my daughter and son)—until the day I die.

About the Author

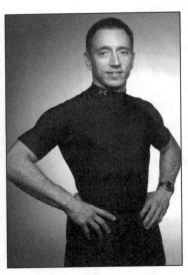

Exercise physiologist, certified personal trainer, and professional speaker, Sal Fichera is a prolific writer, motivational speaker, and media personality whose combination of academic expertise and practical experience makes him uniquely qualified to write about health, fitness, and mind/body synergy.

Fichera is a columnist for *Healthwise* magazine and has written feature articles and editorials, provided expert advice, and evaluated consumer products for publications, including *Cosmopolitan, Good Housekeeping, Fitness Management, New York Times, New York Daily News,* and *The Daily Challenge.*

On the Internet, he has been a consumer-products expert for *WebMd.com, Healthgate.com, Efit.com,* and*My Wellness.com.* He is a source for media professionals who seek his expertise on a wide range of health, fitness, and wellness issues and products, making him a popular and credible go-to guy for everything from holiday health tips to exercising in inclement weather to what is the best exercise equipment. Fichera has made television appearances on *CNN, Dateline NBC, NY1 News,* and has provided commentary for several New York morning news shows, including NBC, ABC, and WB11.

Through seminars, interviews, and workshops, Fichera has earned a reputation for informative presentations that motivate audiences to take actions that can lead to a healthier, more youthful lifestyle. Through a presentation style that is the polar opposite of today's in-your-face infommercial fodder, Sal frames his subject matter and philosophy in a way that empathizes with his audience and gives them the knowledge, skills, structure, and motivation they need to attain success on a personal level. He has lectured on a broad range of health and fitness topics at numerous universities and corporations on the East and West coasts.

Fichera has been studying, practicing, and teaching the benefits of proper exercise and nutrition since 1987. He graduated from St. John's University in Jamaica, New York, with a B.S. in Quantitative Analysis, and he received an M.S. in Exercise Physiology from Queens College (City University of New York). In 1989, Fichera founded Forza Fitness, a company that blends holistic philosophy with cutting-edge scientific research.

Before dedicating his life to the fitness profession, Fichera worked in the corporate realm—first as a software programmer, then as a real estate agent and appraiser, and then as a corporate recruiter. His combination of practical experience and formal education has given him a fully rounded approach to solutions for health and appearance concerns. Quality of life, reversing the biological clock, and becoming leaner, stronger, and healthier . . . that is his focus and therein lies the heart of Sal's dedication to his clients and his audiences.

Sal is currently at work on his next book. He and his wife, Ryoko, live in New York City, and he can be contacted through his website www.ForzaFitness.com.